THE HONEST WEIGH

No diets, no guilt, no calorie counting - just real nutrition, mindset alignment and lifestyle mastery.

Gemma Mullinger

Copyright © 2025 Gemma Mullinger

All rights reserved. No part of this publication may be reproduced, distributed or transmitted in any form or by any means, including photocopying, recording or other electronic or mechanical methods, without the prior permission of the publisher, except in the case of brief quotations embodied in critical reviews and certain other non-commercial uses permitted by copyright law.

Although the author has made every effort to ensure that the information in this book was correct at press time, the author does not assume any liability to any party for any loss, damage, or disruption caused by errors or omissions, whether such errors or omissions result from negligence, accident or any other cause.

The information in this book is provided for informational purposes only, and should not be used to replace the specialist medical advice and professional judgement of a doctor or health care practitioner. The author can not be held responsible for the use of the information provided in this book. Please always consult a trained professional before making any decision regarding treatment of yourself or others.

For everyone who has ever been on a diet, and especially for those who feel as though they have tried them all.

GEMMA MULLINGER

Introduction

Are you trying to lose weight? Do you feel as if you have tried all the diets with no lasting success? Are you looking for a solution once and for all? What would it mean to you to be able to give up diets forever and become your happiest, healthiest self?

My name is Gemma Mullinger, and I almost fell down the diet rabbit hole aged 20, when I weighed just a little bit more than I wanted to and attempted to do something about it. I joined a gym but didn't attend regularly and had no idea what I was doing. I would spend hours on cardio each week with no noticeable results. I had always loved food and came from a family where food was plentiful and celebrated, but I had never been particularly concerned about eating 'healthily'. I was raised on a varied diet, and quite literally would eat anything! Fresh fruit, vegetables, meat and fish were staples, but so were cakes, biscuits, sweets, packaged snacks and desserts, and ultra-processed foods like tinned meatballs and turkey twizzlers. Fortunately, I grew up with absolutely no diet culture in my household, so I wasn't instantly drawn to slimming clubs and fad diets when deciding how I would approach my desire to lose weight. I tried to cut back on the amount of food I was eating, and much of my food shopping consisted of low calorie, ultra-processed products. Initially, I filled my lunchboxes with packets of 'light' snacks and low-fat yoghurts, proudly showing off how 'good' I was being. It didn't work! I tried another gym a few years later, again with no noticeable weight loss, and then, by chance, decided to give group exercise classes a try. With no reliable guidance and conflicting information coming at me from all directions in the media, and from people I knew, it really was a case of 'trial and error'. With the instruction and support that the group exercise sessions provided, I started dropping the pounds, and noticing a change in my physique, fitness and mindset. The classes became just as important for my social wellbeing and stress relief as they were for physical health, but as I was settling into a routine which worked for me, I fell ill and was diagnosed with an inflammatory bowel condition called Ulcerative Colitis. At the time I was a deputy manager at a supermarket – a job which was physically demanding and involved working more than 60 hours a week. Stress, lack of sleep, poor eating habits and working too much had massively contributed to my illness; a condition which cannot be cured, only managed. I almost instantly decided that life was too short to stay in a job which had these implications for my health and happiness, so in a spontaneous move, I started training to be a gym instructor and personal trainer at my local college instead. I had never been sporty, and sports day at school had always been the worst day of the year for me, so my new college course was a huge jump outside of my comfort zone. I didn't question whether it was right for me; it was almost as if it was something I knew I needed to do. Although, looking back, the qualifications were basic and very centred around government guidelines for health and nutrition, I enjoyed the time I spent training, and a spark of passion for all things health and wellness was ignited in me. I lost the weight I wanted to lose, and with the help of lots of additional reading and research, I learnt so much about the principles of nutrition, healthy eating, and weight loss. I started digging deeper into diet culture and educated myself on what behaviours and habits were really needed to lose weight and maintain optimum health, as well as to live a happy life.

My first fitness job was in a ladies only gym; a place where I felt totally comfortable and at home. I felt drawn towards working with women who, like me, were not naturally sporty or interested in exercise. After a year, I made the decision to leave my job and go self-employed. I had no business knowledge or experience, and passion alone was not a strong enough foundation to build a successful business. After 18 months I have up my little fitness studio, returning to retail and the safety of an employed job. Getting pregnant and having my little boy, Cassius, in 2016 was the catalyst for setting up on my own again, and as soon as I could, I was back to running classes, bootcamps and weight loss groups. More than anything, I just wanted to help other women to end their struggles with their weight and enjoy food, fitness and feeling healthy. It was hard with a young baby, and when he started pre-school aged 2, I wanted to make more money during the hours he was being looked after, and to not have to go out in the evenings to work, which was when fitness classes were mostly attended. Cue the introduction of an 'accidental' cleaning business! It was only ever meant to be a bit of extra income for a few hours a week, but it soon became financially successful, and grew to include a team of cleaners, allowing me flexibility and freedom, and the long-awaited feeling that I had finally succeeded in running my own business. Five years later, I was still running that business, but knew I wanted and needed more when it came to my career. I had always been interested in nutrition, but over the last few years that interest had developed into a passion – one which I am now completely absorbed in every single day!

So, here we are in 2025 – I've come full circle and I'm getting stuck back into building a career involving the things in life I love the most – health, wellness, and food! I have been studying for a Masters in Human Nutrition at the University of Plymouth since September 2024, and will graduate towards the end of this year as a fully qualified nutritionist! I have finally taken notice of my purpose and true calling in life. It has been screaming out at me for years, but I've pushed it away, believing that it would be too hard to make a living doing something I loved so much. Every time I did anything in an unrelated industry, I would quickly feel unfulfilled, bored, and desperate to do something more aligned with my true self. I know that I am here to help people to live their healthiest, happiest lives; to share my knowledge and experience with others, and support them to lose weight, love food, and, most importantly, to be the person that they want to become. I feel so fortunate that I discovered a passion for health and wellness when I did, and I'm pretty sure that if I hadn't, I'd probably be struggling with my own weight issues right now.

Eighteen years after my weight loss and wellbeing journey started, I still find myself frustrated and saddened daily by the conflicting information and confusing advice shared with those who want to shed the pounds and become healthier. The biggest benefit of waiting so long to write this book is that the content I share within it has stood the test of time – I've been living by these 18 strategies myself for the last eighteen years. I've managed to continue to indulge my own love of food while maintaining a weight I am happy with and a positive attitude towards eating. I have even managed to heal my digestive health condition using food and lifestyle, despite doctors saying I would always suffer with it. I'd love to share what has worked for me, and some of the knowledge that I have amassed over the years so that others can release themselves from the cycle of frustration, shame and chronic poor health caused by perpetual dieting. I have always wanted to write a book. Writing is my favourite way of sharing what I know with the world, and I absolutely adore books and reading, so this is a real passion project for me.

This book discusses aspects of weight loss which are often missed in diets and healthy eating programmes. You will notice a strong focus on mindset, identity, sustainability, and balance as opposed to strict rules, quick fixes, and unreliable nutrition advice. It has occurred to me during the process of writing this book that I am sharing my beliefs, feelings, and opinions as they stand at the moment of publishing. I am committing what I know and think right now to print, but some things are likely to change in time. Science will become outdated, and how I feel about certain elements of health, wellbeing and weight loss may alter or evolve. With the content of this book, I aim to be as timeless as possible. The principles I share are ones that I know to be true for myself, and I feel that whatever changes in society and science, they will remain integral to how I live my life. It feels good for me to share the content of this book, knowing that I am unlikely to look back on it in another eighteen years and feel that it is no longer useful. I am as sure as I can be that my weight and health will still be supported by these strategies in another decade or two, and yours can be too. I will always be interested in what science has to say, enjoy learning about new research and seeing how advice changes, and I'm really open to listening to others, and changing my views, but you can adopt my strategies now with the confidence that they won't be out of date any time soon.

I'm beyond excited to get this book out there into the hands and onto the e-readers of the people who need it the most. I hope that by writing it and sharing what I know, I will be able to help people to move away from dieting completely, experience improved body positivity, and start to enjoy life and food without worry, obsession, or shame. Nobody wants to spend their whole life on a diet, and I'm so happy that you are here, ready to learn The Honest Weigh and set yourself free from diets, guilt and confusion. This is real nutrition, mindset alignment and lifestyle mastery, and it may even change your life. Enjoy!

Gemma x

Note: Before you start to delve into the rest of this book, I want you to find or buy a notebook which will become a place for you to journal throughout your journey. A space for you to release your feelings and thoughts, a place to make notes should you wish, and to complete the tasks given to you as you move through the strategies that this book delivers.

PHASE 1: TRUTH AND CLARITY

STRATEGY 1: GIVE UP DIETING – FOREVER!

"You deserve to live a life that doesn't revolve around dieting or losing weight" (Unknown)

Another diet is not the answer! I need to start The Honest Weigh by exploring the worrying situation we find ourselves in as a nation when it comes to health and weight, and why giving up dieting is the first step you need to take on your journey to becoming your healthiest, happiest self. This had to be the focus of my first strategy, because I truly believe that if you continue to diet, you will always battle with food and with your weight. A harmonious relationship with both is possible if you can move away from the diet mentality.

With the UK diet industry alone reported to be worth an estimated £2bn annually, and people spending so much of their hard-earned cash on meal plans, programmes, memberships, clubs and apps supposedly designed to help them lose weight, we must start questioning why obesity is more prevalent than it ever has been. Surely, with all the done-for-you diets, supportive communities, and easy to use technologies available, reaching and maintaining your ideal weight should be easier than ever before. But unfortunately, this couldn't be further from reality.

The statistics shared by the UK parliament use the categories 'obese', 'overweight', and 'neither obese or overweight'. The Health Survey for England 2021 disclosed that 63.8%

of British adults are considered to make up the 'obese' and 'overweight' categories, leaving 36.2% who are 'neither obese or overweight'. This means that roughly two thirds of adults in the UK are heavier than it is deemed healthy for them to be. I feel that I need to say at this point that the method used to determine which weight category as individual falls into is questionable to say the least. This debate in itself could be the subject of an entirely separate book! BMI (Body Mass Index) in simple terms, is the relationship between height and weight. There are so many limitations with this method. To some degree, yes, the taller you are, the more you can weigh and avoid being 'overweight' or 'obese'. However, this simple measurement fails to consider all of the other variables which can affect an individual's body composition, such as age, sex, ethnicity, muscle mass, genetics and body shape. It would be hard to assess all of these factors for the purpose of gaining accurate statistics though, and although a hip-waist ratio has been hailed as a more appropriate measurement to base research on, it could also be argued that weight shouldn't always be a deciding factor as to whether a person is healthy or not.

What do you think? Can a person who is overweight be considered healthy? What if they are healthy in all other areas, but are still carrying extra weight? Would this even be considered as 'extra' weight is they were healthy in every other way? Or, do you believe that is this person was *truly* healthy, they wouldn't be overweight in the first place? I don't think there are any hard and fast answers here. This hypothetical dilemma shows that health is a concept which is much more complex than you might initially think, and it can be defined in many ways – 'one size fits all' definitely does not apply here: quite literally!

Regardless of how we take the measurements, what we base our statistics on, and how we define health, there is no escaping the fact that there *is* an increase in the amount of people struggling with their weight. Some of these people may indeed consider themselves to be healthy despite this, but many will not. So, why are we dealing with this rise in rates of obesity and being overweight?

If we look back to The National Heights and Weights Survey of 1980, just 9% of women and 6% of men were affected by obesity, and in the 1960s it was even rarer. It seems that changes in lifestyle since the eighties have caused more people to struggle with obesity and being overweight. The introduction of supermarkets, fast food outlets, desk jobs, microwaves, ready meals, and more ultra-processed food, combined with an increase in sugar consumption, and more time sitting down for entertainment purposes have all had a combined and catastrophic impact on the weight and health of people in our society. And, instead of using what we know about these changes to look at how we could make things better, society has turned in its droves to diets, diets, and more diets!

Dieting doesn't work. This is my opinion, anyway, but the statistic that is often thrown around states that 97% of diets fail. In reality, it would be impossible to know the truth about how many of the people embarking on diets actually manage to lose weight, and furthermore maintain the loss over time. However, the increasing prevalence of obesity within society suggests that attempts to find a solution are rarely successful. Before thinking about how we can manage out weight and health, we are going to consider the reasons why dieting doesn't often work, and the negative effects it can have on your physical and mental health.

Would you go to a clothes shop to buy a pair of trousers, find a pair you like and buy the first pair from the rail without checking the size? Would you buy a pair in a size 10 just because your friend wears a size 10 and she looks great in them, even though you normally wear a size 16? No! Most people sign up or commit to diets in this way, though. There are many different weight loss methods on the market today. Among them, programmes, plans, pills, injections, apps, groups, detoxes and diets. Perhaps the most crucial reason these offerings often fail is that they do not consider individual requirements, preferences, lifestyle, and importantly, the *reason* why someone became overweight in the first place. Many diets are written and marketed by individuals who have previously struggled with their own weight. The diet they sell is based on what worked for them, and there is no guarantee that this will also work for anyone else who decides to follow it.

Eating a healthy, balanced diet certainly does not have to mean eating boring and bland food, but going 'on a diet' instantly makes most people think of the things they will have to cut out, and how miserable it will make them. A diet may involve limiting your intake of certain foods, reducing calorie consumption in general, or a combination of both. People setting out to lose weight often pledge to avoid the foods they love the most, which only exacerbates the feeling that going on a diet will result in unhappiness! The natural response to deprivation is to want something even more. So, when, in an attempt to lose weight, you ban yourself from consuming certain foods and drinks, or reduce your overall intake of food drastically, it is inevitable that you will want to eat and drink even more. Eventually, your initial willpower will fade, and you will succumb to the food or drink that you have desperately missed, likely consuming an intake greater than it would have been, had you allowed yourself to eat or drink it without restriction. Cutting out certain foods completely without good reason, and excessively reducing calories are not sustainable actions and will not help you with weight management in the long term.

In your head, it's *not* for the long term though. This is part of the problem. A diet is a set of instructions which you intend to follow for a short, sometimes defined, period of time. When you set out on your diet, it is likely that you will already have the end in mind – that moment where you can treat yourself for losing weight by visiting your favourite cake shop, ordering a takeaway, or enjoying the sweets and chocolates you missed so much while you were dieting. By treating your health and weight management as a short term 'problem' that you *must* deal with, rather than a lifestyle which you *want* to nurture, you will struggle to achieve results which last longer than a few weeks or months. This then creates a cycle whereby you want to lose weight, so you try a diet, it doesn't work as you had hoped, so you stop. You are still unhappy with your weight, so at some point in the future you decide to try again, or try a different diet, and the same thing happens. The more diets you try, the more disordered your eating and your relationship with food becomes. It is an accumulative effect, and you become more and more indoctrinated by diet culture, diet rules and diet mentality. A healthy relationship with food becomes a distant memory; one which is hard to recover.

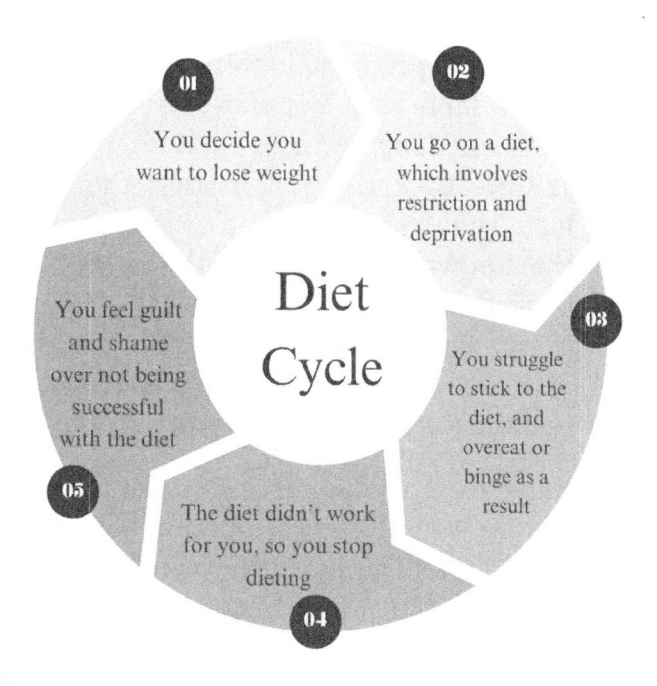

Diet Cycle

01 You decide you want to lose weight

02 You go on a diet, which involves restriction and deprivation

03 You struggle to stick to the diet, and overeat or binge as a result

04 The diet didn't work for you, so you stop dieting

05 You feel guilt and shame over not being successful with the diet

Dieting slowly chips away at your own inbuilt ability to eat intuitively – something we will delve into more deeply later. Being on a diet causes you to rely on the directions given to you, and as a result alters the process involved in choosing food and deciding on portion sizes. While this might be effective for the duration of the diet, as soon as you decide to relax the rules, the weight loss slows down, stops or even reverses because you become reliant on having your food intake dictated by the principles of the diet you were following. In other words, you literally don't know what food to choose for yourself anymore! This is why some people who join slimming clubs or follow large scale popular diets decide to stay on them long term so that they can avoid gaining back the weight that they initially lost. They are dependent, and unable to stop the diet whilst keeping off the weight, so they trick themselves into believing that staying on the diet is a 'healthy lifestyle' The cult-like approach of these clubs only encourages this mentality even more.

Diets are not only terrible at getting you the lasting weight loss results that you want, but they can also be harmful to your physical and mental health. Some of the consequences you may experience are listed below:

- Nutrient deficiencies
- Digestive issues
- Loss of muscle mass
- Disturbances of your menstrual cycle
- Fatigue/tiredness
- Reduced bone density
- Mood problems
- Depression and/or anxiety
- Difficulty concentrating/brain fog
- Developing a poor relationship with food (and potential for eating disorders)
- Slower metabolism
- Gut dysbiosis
- Increase in stress hormone (cortisol) production

Finally, we come to the inspiration for this book – the reality that most diets and weight loss methods focus solely on food and exercise; failing to address the important matter of mindset, and the implications that it can have on health and weight management. The concepts I share within this book recognise the importance of food and movement, but also concentrate on encouraging you to think differently, change your mindset, consider the person you would like to become, take responsibility for your own weight and health, and utilise non-diet ways to help you to lose weight and become healthier.

Despite their ineffectiveness and potential for side effects, there are countless options when it comes to diets, each with their own attraction points and pitfalls. By briefly discussing a few common types of diet, I hope to help you to realise that if you want to lose weight and improve your health, there must be a better way than opting for yet another diet, regardless of which one you might have chosen.

Let's first think about calorie counting. It's a very simple concept, which involves tracking the number of calories in the foods you consume and making sure that they don't exceed a set amount. This figure is often decided upon because it is lower than the number of calories you would be likely to burn in an average day, therefore causing a calorie deficit, which should, in theory, lead to weight loss. This *can* give good weight loss results initially, simply because you are making a change to the way you are normally eating. Your 'required' calorie intake is based on several factors, including your gender, size, age, and activity levels, so if you *were* to follow a calorie-controlled diet, your upper limit would need to be determined individually. Low calorie (800-1500) and very low calorie (800 or fewer) diets can have unpleasant and dangerous side effects including fatigue, nutrient deficiencies, headaches, nausea, and even infertility. When I typed '1200 calorie diet' into an internet search engine, I was surprised to see that well-known organisations claiming to care about health had webpages sharing these kinds of diets, even though having a calorie intake this low is unhealthy for most people. Not eating enough calories can also cause metabolism to slow down, thus having a detrimental effect on weight loss. Recent research has also shown that the simple 'calories in must be less than calories out' equation for weight loss may not even be reliable, as the gut microbiota has an impact on how this works in different individuals. The calorie content shown on food packaging may not be the amount actually absorbed by the body, and this can vary greatly between individuals. What seems like a simple weight loss tool becomes a lot more complicated when you consider all of these factors! Perhaps the biggest problem with calorie counting, in my opinion, is that many dieters completely disregard the nutritional content of their food and focus their concern only on staying within their calorie limit, therefore prioritising weight loss above overall health. Calories are simply a measure of how much energy your food contains, not a measure of nutrition, food quality or how that food might affect you as an individual. Dr Tim Spector, a well-known medical doctor and science writer, says that with very strict calorie counting you may lose some weight for a few weeks but "even if you are successful, your body's evolutionary mechanisms make you hungrier and hungrier every week you go by when you're depriving yourself of energy". Your body goes into shutdown mode to reserve as much energy as possible because it feels threatened by the reduction in calories. However, calorie-controlled diets are often the 'go-to' for those wanting to lose weight, and are still regularly promoted by coaches, fitness instructors, health professionals, and health organisations as a good way to do so.

Similarly, there are a range of point counting diets, which, as the name suggests, require the follow to adhere to a set number of points rather than calories One well-known slimming club allocates members 15 'Syns' daily, allowing them to include a limited amount of specified foods in their diet which are deemed not to be conducive to weight loss. Upon carrying out some research into 'Syns' online, I discovered that there were many websites listing popular snacks and sweets which are considered to be 'low Syn'. These included things like a Mars Bar (6 Syns), Options Belgian Hot Chocolate (2 Syns), Curly Wurly Bar (3 Syns) and Oreo Thins (1.5 Syns per biscuit). These foods are all ultra-processed, contain high amounts of sugar or artificial sweeteners, and other ingredients which could have a negative effect on your health. Meanwhile, a tablespoon of double cream comes in at 3.5 Syns, 100g of mushrooms cooked in oil or butter racks up 7 Syns, and 25g of Brazil nuts uses 8.5 Syns! You can see how this way of eating could easily encourage dieters to choose ultra-processed foods instead of ingredients which are perfectly healthy and balanced. Many people who are coming from a place of struggling with food and with their weight would struggle to choose a small handful of nuts over a Mars Bar and a hot chocolate, both of which they could have for less than the number of Syns contained in the nuts! Point counting diets have similar flaws to calorie counting diets, in that they encourage followers to use numbers to decide what to eat, rather than their own intuition, emotions and more detailed information about the nutritional content of the food. As previously mentioned, these diets often have a cult-like feel, and a big social support element, so followers could be tempted to stay on them for longer or return to them even if they didn't really work before. It might sound dramatic, but I believe these diets have the potential to be quite dangerous; both physically and mentally.

Moving on, let's look at low-fat diets. Low-fat diets first became popular in America in the 1960s, when research linked saturated fat to heart disease. It is thought by some that this research was commissioned by the sugar industry, who wanted to shift the blame for poor heart health away from sugar in order to protect their profits. As a result, fat was demonised, and low-fat diet were recommended by doctors to those with elevated risk of cardiovascular disease. By the 1980s, this advice had transmuted to the general population, and after seeing the low-fat approach promoted by the government, health service, doctors and food manufacturers, a large percentage of the population started to follow it. Although we now know that the recommendation was not healthy or helpful for the vast majority, choosing low-fat foods became a way of life for many, and a hard belief to shake off. When I first started working in the health and fitness industry back in 2013, most of my clients consciously chose low-fat foods because they believed they were healthier, and some showed genuine panic when I recommended that they move towards full-fat products. Low-fat diets are very detrimental to your health and wellbeing, with potential side effects including poor brain function, hormonal imbalance, vitamin deficiency and malabsorption, dry skin, hair loss and depression.

Keto and paleo type diets are very popular currently. The diets have a lot of similarities, with the main features of both being a high intake of fat and limited carbohydrates. Keto aims to get the body into a state of ketosis, where there is no glucose to burn for energy, causing the body to burn fat from stores in the body instead. Paleo focuses on eliminating processed foods and emulating the diet of people in The Stone Age. Both can have health weight loss benefits, and there are elements of each diet which make good nutritional sense – in fact, these diets are probably closest to the way I choose to eat. However, when followed strictly for a long time can come with a list of possible side effects, including bad breath, skin rashes, headaches, lethargy, digestive disturbances and mood swings. With keto, it would be challenging to maintain any results obtained if you returned to pre-keto behaviours. Neither diet is easy to stick to and can feel restrictive. The main problem with this type of diet is that they are extreme and come with a lot of strict rules. While I value the health benefits from these diets, I would struggle to commit to the strictness required – never eating carbohydrates or any ingredients not considered Paleo ever again. This is why I don't give my way of eating a name or tie myself to a specific type of diet.

Intermittent fasting, meaning that you don't eat for a specified period each day or week, has gained popularity over recent years. Giving your body an extended break from digesting food is thought to benefit heart health, reduce the risk of Type 2 diabetes, and decrease inflammation in the body. Having fewer hours in which you can eat naturally reduces your calorie intake too, meaning that weight loss is also hailed as a benefit. Essentially, intermittent fasting could be viewed as an alternative way to follow a calorie-controlled diet. In the UK, Micheal Mosley's 2012 BBC documentary 'Eat, Fast and Live Longer' brought intermittent fasting – in particular the

5:2 diet – to the forefront of the diet industry. There are different ways to incorporate fasting into your lifestyle. The 5:2 diet involves eating as you usually would for 5 days, and reducing calories to 500-600 on each of the remaining 2 days of the week, whereas the 16:8 gives you an 8 hour window in which to eat, and the remaining 16 hours of the day are spent fasting. Regardless of the science behind this kind of diet, my first concern is that deliberately depriving yourself during specified hours or days may affect the amount of food you eat and the choices you make when you are 'allowed to eat as normal'. I also think that the language used when describing and marketing these diets is a problem, with phrases like 'eat normally for 5 days' or 'eat a healthy, balanced diet for 5 days and restrict your eating for 2'. What does 'eating normally' mean? What does a 'healthy, balanced diet' mean? And by using the word 'restrict', it is implied that deprivation is needed to reach and sustain a healthy weight. There are undoubtedly some benefits that can be enjoyed with intermittent fasting, but as with all weight loss methods, only if it suits your lifestyle and comes naturally rather than feeling forced as part of a diet.

Finally, I want to touch upon meal plans, which involve simply following a set plan which has been provided for you. These are different from the meal planning that you do for yourself, which can be a really helpful part of a healthy lifestyle. Meal plans vary from simple plans shared in magazines and newspapers, often based on calorie counting or a low-fat diet, to individualised plans designed by personal trainers or nutritionists. Plans like these will vary greatly in success, but ultimately, they cause reliance upon being told what to eat, and interfere with natural intuition around food. Meal plans are often restrictive, in that they do not always take into consideration the preferences , dietary requirements, lifestyle commitments, cooking ability and budget of the user. Even a well thought out meal plan written by a qualified nutritionist causes reliance on the meal planning service. They my work as a quick fix, but never as a long-term solution to weight struggles, unless you plan on paying for the services of the nutritionist indefinitely. Even if you *did* do this, your reliance on the meal plans could prove problematic in terms of your happiness and relationship with food.

I have briefly discussed a few types of diets, but there are thousands more specifically named diets available to people wanting to lose weight – when I did an online search, the results included, but were definitely not limited to: The Blood Type Diet, Zone Diet, DASH Diet, Beverly Hills Diet, Cabbage Soup Diet, Baby Food Diet, Alkaline Diet, Celery Juice Diet, Atkins Diet, Dukan Diet, Fast 800 Diet, The Low GI Diet, Macrobiotic Diet, South Beach

Diet, Raw Diet, Body For Life, Nutrisystem, and even The Cookie Diet!

None of the above types of diet look at the root cause of your weight struggles, offer any support with motivation or inspiration, or prompt you to think about how your mindset could be impacting your weight. Remember that health is holistic, meaning that we should consider the whole person when assessing health or looking for ways to make improvements. This could include physical factors such as nutrition, movement and sleep, emotional factors like grief or loneliness, mental health considerations such as anxiety and depression, financial matters, spirituality and more. Diets will often focus solely on food, and many programmes or plans will cover food *and* fitness, but most will neglect areas like emotions, sources of motivation, your upbringing, and impact of underlying beliefs. That is why the principles shared in this book are based less on what you need to eat and what exercises to do, and more on learning what works for you, your mindset, identity, lifestyle, and attitude. I believe that The Honest Weigh can really help you to achieve success in your weight loss journey, and in your long-term healthy lifestyle, but this book will not have all the information you need. Depending on your circumstances, interests, current health situation and your journey so far, you may need additional resources and support in areas like hormonal health, nutrition for specific health conditions, eating disorders, body positivity, being healthy on a budget, bringing up healthy children, and more. There are some fantastic health books, podcasts, and social media accounts available to you, and I absolutely believe that you should access these if you feel called to do so.

If you are to succeed in losing weight and maintaining your ideal weight, you must become comfortable with the fact that there is no 'magic pill'! Dr Chris Van Tulleken shares in his book 'Ultra-Processed People' his opinion that individuals who have experienced long-term obesity need to take weight loss drugs or have surgery in order to lose weight and keep it off. I don't share this belief. In my time as a health and fitness professional, I have met people who have tried all the diets, taken weight loss pharmaceuticals, and even some who have had bariatric surgery. Losing weight and maintaining a healthy weight is something which requires lifelong consideration and input. A six-week diet, one-time surgery, or repeat prescription of a weight loss drug will not be good enough to replace this – no matter how effective it was for you initially. As you decide to stop dieting, you will also need to make a mindset shift away from the 'magic pill' mentality, and the thought that there may just be something out there that will offer you a quick and easy solution.

Finally, don't be brainwashed! An important element of The Honest Weigh is the corruption and coercion within the diet and food industries. I want to encourage you to understand that companies, brands, influencers, and ambassadors often release and promote diets and diet-related products with the primary goal of making money. If a diet worked long-term, the consumer would no longer need to pay for the product, and therefore there needs to be an element of reliable in order to obtain repeat business and for profits to continue. There is little money to be made in the diet and weight loss industry from healthy, slim people who can maintain their own weight and health. Thinking about the previously mentioned points diet allowing followers 15 'Syns' a day, you have to question why people need to keep returning to meetings for years on end if it is supposedly so successful. Why aren't these followers losing weight and keeping it off? Consider where you are choosing to spend your money, what you get in return, and how the companies or individuals benefit from you purchasing their goods or services. Do they really want you to succeed?

I want to open your eyes to what is possible for you. I want to help you to understand how good you are capable of feeling. I feel excited to take you on this journey of freedom and discovery to your healthiest, happiest self, but before we move on, I'd like you to take some time to complete the task below. Don't be tempted to rush through this – block out an hour of uninterrupted time where you can really consider your answer to each question.

Task:

Get out your diary and journal on the questions below.

Which diets have you tried in the past? You may want to write about each one on a separate page, so that you have space to answer the following questions with each diet in mind.
1. **How did each diet make you feel?**
2. **What results did you have, and how long did these results last?**
3. **Why did you stop each diet?**
4. **What happened afterwards?**
5. **Would you try the diet again? If so, why? If not, why not?**

Collectively, what does this information tell you about how diets make you feel, the effect they have on your physical and mental health, and their success rate for you personally?

Do you feel ready to change your way of thinking so that you can say goodbye to dieting for good?

Considering the content you have read so far; how do you feel about continuing to read and implement this book?

GEMMA MULLINGER

How would you like to feel after you have finished reading it?
What impact do you expect this book to have on your health and happiness?

Strategy Summary:

- If you continue to diet, I believe you will always struggle with your weight.
- The diet industry is worth around £2bn annually in the UK, but over two thirds of adults are classed as overweight or obese.
- Obesity was rare in the 1960s, and the rates have risen sharply since the 1980s. Our lifestyle and the food we eat are to blame!
- Diets are 'one size fits all', short term and restrictive. They can affect your mindset, and can cause a range of nasty side effects, both mental and physical.
- Most diets are extreme rather than balanced, and this means that they can be hard to stick to and can be unhealthy.
- There is no magic pill when it comes to weight loss!

STRATEGY 2: LIVE A HEALTHY LIFSTYLE – IT REALLY IS THAT SIMPLE!

"Sorry, there's no magic bullet. You gotta eat healthily and live healthy to be healthy and look health. End of story". (Morgan Spurlock)

"If dieting isn't the way forward, then what should we do instead?" I hear you ask! Well, in short, the answer is 'a long-term healthy lifestyle'. Yes, it really is that simple! However, simple does not mean *easy*. If achieving a healthy lifestyle was easy, there wouldn't be so many people struggling with their weight in the first place, and turning to diets out of desperation. If it was that easy, I'd be finishing the book right here! Of course, what you want to know now is *how* to create that healthy lifestyle in order to achieve the results you are keen to see. What does this healthy lifestyle look like? It all sounds a little bit vague, doesn't it? I want to be honest and upfront with you about what I feel it takes to maintain a weight that you are happy with. Although I am encouraging you not to diet, I am not saying that you won't need to make changes, and these changes can be hard work. What these changes are and how you will approach them is individual and down to you to decide. I can't tell you exactly what a healthy, balanced lifestyle looks like, because everyone has a different version. The remainder of this book will guide you in creating your own healthy, balanced lifestyle, naturally, in a way which suits you and feels enjoyable. I won't be telling you what to eat or what exercise to do. Instead, I aim to help you by providing a collection of interesting, thought provoking, and immediately actionable strategies which will help you to change your

mindset, ultimately making the process more easily achievable and sustainable.

This book comprises a collection of 20 strategies to help you to lose weight and become healthier. Work with The Honest Weigh in any way you choose – follow it in the order it is written or choose to read the strategies that appeal to you first. I have written the book in an order which makes sense to me, and which I feel will be useful to the reader, but I always like to promote individuality and encourage people to do what feels right for them. If a strategy doesn't feel applicable to you, or doesn't resonate, simply skip it!

In Strategy 1, I explained why diets are not usually good for you, and very rarely work in the long term. This may be a concept that you were already aware of and believe in, or it may be completely new to you. You will have spent some time at the end of that strategy journalling around your own history with dieting. Thinking back over the diets you have tried may have brought to the forefront of your mind how you feel in general about diets, and the effect they have on you and your life. Try to remember these feelings as you work through this journey. When things get hard it can be easy to revert back to old habits, and it may seem tempting to start another diet to shed weight quickly rather than reading this book to the end and engaging in the tasks I have set. Some

THE HONEST WEIGH

of the strategies or tasks may challenge you and require more effort than simply reading the words I have written and taking on board what I have to say. If at any point you are considering starting another diet, remember that if any of the diets you had previously tried had worked for you as you wanted them to, you would be maintaining your ideal weight right now. As you continue to read this book, I hope that you will gain confidence in your own intuition and ability, and that you can start to make sustainable, balanced changes to your relationship with food, your eating habits, and your lifestyle in order to become healthier and happier – for good. I hope that you will learn so much from the contents of this book that by the end you will believe as strongly as I do that a healthy, balanced lifestyle is the best way forward. I hope that you will never look back!

Task:

Get out your diary and journal on the questions below.

1. **What do you think a 'healthy, balanced lifestyle' means to you? Don't think too hard about this – just journal around what comes to mind.**

2. **Why do you think you struggle to sustain that lifestyle currently?**

3. **Describe a healthy, balanced lifestyle**

that you feel you would be able to maintain indefinitely.

4. What stops you from living like this already?

'Ultra-processed food' is a phrase you may have heard thrown around in the health and weight loss arena – especially recently! The definition of 'ultra-processed' varies between individuals and organisations, and it can be confusing, especially when considered in relation to processed foods in general. 'Ultra-processed foods are highly altered and typically contain a lot of added salt, sugar, fat, and industrial chemical additives' says Zoe Science and Nutrition. They go on to describe processed foods as those which have had fat, sugar, salt, or oil, and other culinary ingredients added, but are not harmful to our health. Minimally processed or unprocessed foods are those which have not been altered at all or have had no ingredients added. They may have undergone a process to make them edible or easier to store and use, but their nutritional content has not changed. Most of the foods we eat are processed to some extent – yoghurt is fermented milk, peas are frozen to keep them fresh until you eat them, and beans and chickpeas are canned to preserve them. Peanut butter is made by blitzing peanuts until they form a paste, and nutritious dark chocolate goes through many processes before it is edible! Processed foods are not inherently bad for you, but ultra-processed foods can cause a negative effect on your health, particularly when consumed in excess. Ultra-processed foods (UPF) are thought to cause increased rates of obesity, cancer, heart disease, metabolic disease, mental illnesses, and other health conditions. Perhaps the increase in consumption of UPF over the last few decades has contributed to the noticeable increase in prevalence of these problems? Studies have shown that on average, over 60% of a person's diet in the UK is comprised of ultra-processed foods. Shockingly and sadly, this figure is usually higher for children, reaching around 80%. These statistics genuinely worry me, and I feel particularly concerned for the future health of the children whose diets are predominantly made up of UPF.

Dr Chris Van Tulleken's book 'Ultra-Processed People' comes with the tagline 'why do we all eat stuff that isn't food...and why can't we stop?'. Good question, Dr Chris! Ultra-processed foods are *deliberately* designed to be addictive and highly palatable, so by indulging in them it is likely that we will want to eat more – the start of a vicious cycle which becomes harder to break the more you eat. These foods are cheap, readily available, long-lasting, easy to store, presented in 'attractive' packaging, easy to buy, prepare and eat. With the busy lifestyles of today, these foods often win over whole foods, which can be more expensive, have a shorter shelf life, and require much more time and effort to turn into something edible. Do you think that the manufacturers of these ultra-processed foods would allow their families to consume them? I heard a story recently about the late Steve Jobs, founder of Apple, and how he didn't let his children have smartphones or tablets until they were much older. It made me think about why. This was his own product, that he was selling at massively high volumes to children and adults all over the world, making a very large profit, but he wouldn't allow his own children to use them. He knew that his devices were designed to be addictive, and that this would have undesirable effects on a child's physical and mental development. I would bet that the founders and CEOs of companies selling ultra-processed foods would not allow their own children to eat them, as they know the dangers and the processes involved in making them.

The antithesis of ultra-processed foods are whole foods – foods which are in their natural state, or as close to it as possible in order to remain or become edible. Many doctors and nutritionists have said that a good way to detect an ultra-processed food is to read the label and see if it contains any ingredients which you wouldn't have at home in your kitchen. Although 'ultra-processed' is a current buzzword, keeping ultra-processed foods to a minimum and opting for whole foods where possible has been my intention since becoming interested in health and wellbeing 18 years ago. I make as many meals and snacks from scratch as possible, using natural ingredients. When buying food, I make use of local farms for milk, butter, and eggs, go to the butchers for most of the meat I buy, and opt for organic fruit and vegetables where possible. We even buy our flour from a farm just around the corner from our house, where they use shire horses to work the fields where ancient grains grow, producing fabulous wholemeal flour which is naturally low in gluten and high in protein, and completely free from unnecessary treatments, chemicals, or processing other than grinding. I do still visit the supermarket weekly, but bypass what feels like 90% of the products on offer, knowing that they will not support our health, or make us feel good. Looking back on how easily I have maintained my weight and how healthy I have been, I think that this approach has served me well!

Keep ultra-processed foods to a minimum, but don't feel as though you must eradicate them from your diet altogether or feel bad if you do eat them on occasion. Eat the foods that feel good to you, considering the effects they will have on your health, rather than whether you think they will help you to lose weight. As an example, avocados are notoriously high in calories and fat, and some diets and programmes advise against eating them for this reason. However, they are *so* nutritious, and personally I always feel good when I eat avocado, so I choose them often. Similarly, rice cakes are often recommended in diet plans as they are low in calories, but they also contain minimal nutrition, and you also may find them bland and unsatisfying, making them a less than ideal choice! Of course, there are going to be times where you feel that the food choices presented to you won't necessarily have a positive impact on your physical health, but that the enjoyment you will get from them will contribute to social and emotional health, and this, on occasion, outweighs the need for always eating foods which are exceptionally nourishing. For example, tucking into a buffet at a birthday party, knowing that the food has been chosen to please the crowds and not for health reasons, but thoroughly enjoying the occasion.

I think that the key to minimising ultra-processed foods within your diet, and that of your children if you have them, is to get creative with food, and make delicious meals and snacks using whole foods and natural ingredients – this will keep you all satisfied, interested in the food you are eating, and feeling good as a result of what you consume. One of the biggest mistakes people tend to make, in my opinion, when moving away from ultra-processed foods, is to be restrictive, taking on the mentality that whole foods are boring and not varied enough. Naturally, if you are reducing your intake of one thing, you will usually need to replace it with something else. The reduction of ultra-processed foods should be accompanied with an increase in whole foods. This will create the sweet spot where you will start to feel better, notice changes in your health, and not feel as though you are being deprived, because you are still eating plenty of varied and delicious foods. There has been great debate in recent years over the inclusion of animal products in a healthy diet, but I strongly believe that foods like meat, fish, eggs, cheese, butter, yoghurt, and kefir all absolutely have their place within a nutritious, balanced diet, and can have positive health effects for most people. I have always naturally been drawn towards variety, searching for new foods and recipes to try, and ensuring that my meal plan for the week ahead is completely different to the last. Being interested in food and wanting to spend time cooking makes eating whole foods so much easier to achieve. Here are my best tips for improving diversity of whole foods within your nutrition:

- Ask yourself as you browse each section of the supermarket or place where you are shopping, 'what have I not eaten in a long time' and buy that! This works particularly well in the fruit and vegetable aisles, as there are so many different types that you would never be able to take them all home every week. If it crosses your mind that you have not bought an aubergine or kiwi fruit for a long time, pop them in the trolley! Try to consider seasonal produce though, as this will be more budget-friendly, nutritious, better for the environment, and much tastier!

- Use cookbooks, magazines, social media pages, and websites to source new and interesting recipes to try.
- Plan your meals for the week ahead so that you can make sure you have enough diversity across the 7 days. Ask your family to get involved, as they may come up with ideas that you wouldn't have thought of, and you are more likely to have clean plates if they have helped you to choose what is on the menu!
- Ask your friends for their favourite nutritious recipes – the ones they go back to again and again because they are so good! I once posted a status on Facebook asking for recipe recommendations and received so many new ideas to try.
- Try to choose recipes from different cultures – you'll find that this encourages you to include ingredients that you may not normally choose, for example, harissa, tahini, turmeric, or pomegranate. This helps to vary the nutrients within

your meal, as well as keeping it interesting.

Task:

List as many ultra-processed foods that you can think of that you currently eat regularly.

For each of the above foods, try to think of a whole food-based alternative which could provide a similar eating experience. For example, swapping boxed cereal for a homemade granola or eggs and avocado, milk chocolate for a high cocoa content dark chocolate, shop bought desserts for homemade fruit crumble and cream, and that mid-afternoon biscuit for a sliced apple with peanut butter.

Take a look at the packaging of some of the ultra-processed foods that you currently eat a lot of. Spend 10-20 minutes using the internet to research the impact that some of these ingredients could have on your health and weight. Look at ingredients like aspartame, sucralose, high fructose corn syrup, monosodium glutamate (MSG, and others.

Journal around your thoughts and feelings as you discover the contents of the foods you eat regularly. Does it make you feel that you want to consume less of these foods, knowing how impactful they could be to your health and weight?

Strategy Summary:

- Always aim for a healthy, balanced lifestyle instead of dieting.
- Everyone has their own version of a healthy, balanced lifestyle.
- You may get tempted to revert to dieting when things feel hard or if you are not noticing the results you want. On these occasions, try to remember how dieting made you feel and that if it had worked for you in the past, you would be at your preferred weight right now.
- While many foods available to us have been processed, we should be concerned about our intake of ultra-processed foods – those which have undergone industrial processes and/or include industrial additives like dyes, flavour enhancers, emulsifiers, and stabilisers.
- The average person in the UK has a diet made up of over 60% ultra-processed foods. This figure is higher for children.
- Ultra-processed foods have been linked to increased risk of obesity, cancer, heart disease, diabetes, and other health conditions.
- As important as reducing ultra-processed foods is increasing the diversity of the whole foods you are eating. This increases the range of nutrients your body will

benefit from, and make it less likely that you will become bored of what you are eating.

STRATEGY 3: WORK OUT THE ROOT CAUSE.

"When solving problems, dig at the roots instead of just hacking at the leaves". (Anthony J. D'Angelo)

If you visit the doctor with a sore throat, he or she will try to determine whether it has been caused by a bacterial infection or a virus, in order to know whether to prescribe antibiotics. For a bacterial infection these may be necessary to clear the infection and help you to feel better, but for a virus, they will have no effect at all. Taking antibiotics without good cause could have negative effects on your health, so it is vital to first find the root cause of your symptoms. I think this analogy applied nicely to weight loss, too. As the opening quote for this strategy alludes to, without knowing the reason why a problem has occurred, your attempts to solve that problem will just be a stab in the dark. You will always be stuck in a perpetual cycle of dieting if you do not work with the root cause of your weight struggles. To really be able to work at solving the issue of weighing more than you would like, it can be helpful to identify the root cause of your weight gain. The root cause is an initial occurrence, situation or circumstance which initiated your weight gain and caused a struggle in losing it again. This could be a one-off event like pregnancy weight gain or a bereavement which triggered unhealthy emotional eating patterns, a long-term causative factor such as medication or menopause, or an accumulation of factors over a period of time.

To be able to start to work out the best way forward, you'll need to be able to discover when you started to gain weight, why this happened, and the reasons why you have not been able to lose weight or maintain weight loss for any length of time. The timeline task at the end of this strategy will help you with this.

But firstly, let's look at some of the factors that can cause or contribute towards weight gain.

- Eating/drinking too much
- Eating/drinking too much of certain types of food/drink
- Not achieving enough nutrition in your food intake
- Eating poor quality foods/ultra processed foods
- Not eating enough whole foods
- An unhealthy attitude towards food
- Disordered eating
- Lack of physical activity
- Poor sleep quality/not enough sleep
- Stress
- Trauma
- Unhealthy mindset around food and dieting
- Illness/injury/disability
- Medication
- Family history and genetics
- Hormones (puberty, menstrual cycle, pregnancy and post-partum, peri-menopause, menopause)

Most diets do not consider the root cause of your weight gain, or any individual requirements. A keto diet, for example, could be really damaging for a person with already disordered eating, and a low-calorie diet for someone who already eats very little would be pretty pointless! The first thing you can do to help yourself to become forever free from dieting is to play detective and work out *why* you are overweight, and what the contributing factors have been from birth to the present day.

Task:
You may think you already know the reason for your weight struggles, but I want you to do this exercise anyway. You never know what you might uncover.

Using the blank timeline, start to plot in life events, including things like starting school, moving to a new school, going to college, parents separating, starting university, getting your first job, a new relationship, a relationship ending, pregnancy, marriage etc. Add anything which you feel has been influential on your weight, health or happiness, big or small.

Now look back over the timeline of your life, from the beginning, and if you can, mark the point where you very first started to gain weight. Continuing along the timeline, mark the occasions where you have lost or gained weight

When you have finished, journal around the following questions, using your timeline as a prompt.

1. Can you pinpoint when you very first started to gain weight?
2. What is the reason, behaviour, event or circumstance that triggered your weight gain initially?
3. Why do you think that this happened?
4. Looking back, how does this make you feel now?
5. Since starting to gain weight, have you remained consistently overweight, or have there been times where you have returned to a weight you have been happy with?
6. What do you think triggered or contributed to weight loss over the course of your timeline?
7. What do you think has caused or contributed to your most recent weight gain?
8. Across your whole timeline, what behaviours do you think have caused you to remain overweight, gain weight back again after losing it, or struggle to maintain a loss?
9. Are there any patterns you can notice – reasons for weight loss or weight gain which occur more than once?

THE HONEST WEIGH

Write everything down and be totally honest, giving as much detail as possible.

Timeline of Your Life

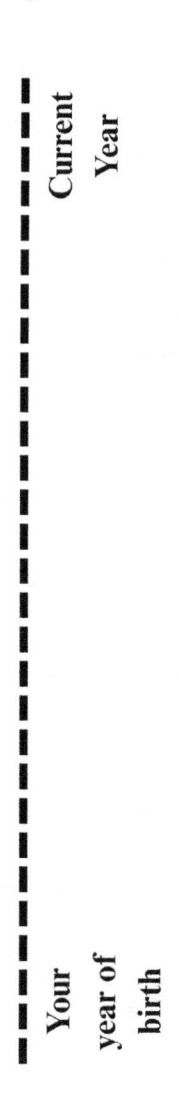

Your year of birth

Current Year

You should now have a much clearer idea of how you got to be where you are with your weight currently. This story is unique to you, and therefore needs a unique solution – which is unlikely to come in the form of a diet and is much more likely to be found in a long-term healthy lifestyle, as suggested in the previous strategy. When you have discovered the root cause(s) for your weight situation, you will then need to do your own further research into how you can help yourself to overcome those problems, or minimise the effects of them. I would never be able to cover all of them in sufficient detail in this book, and every story is different, so will require a different approach. It is important that you take responsibility for your situation and for finding the solution that is right for you. You may need to seek specialist or specific advice or information, in the form of professional support or information from books or reliable online sources.

When I have used the timeline technique with coaching clients, they have been shocked at how looking back over their lives can reveal so much about their relationship with food and with themselves, and about their struggles with losing weight. Almost every time, the client has cried. Doing this involves looking back at hard times in their lives, or times where a lot of changes happened. Recognising that these times have had an impact on their health and happiness can be upsetting but also expansive. I don't like seeing people upset, but this is one of my favourite parts of the coaching that I do, as it always seems to be a moment of revelation and a turning point for my clients in their journey towards understanding themselves better. This is the work that is so desperately needed when it comes to weight loss and living more healthily, but is so often completely ignored in diets and other weight loss programmes, usually in favour of cutting calories, restricting certain foods, and a more aesthetic focused approach.

The fictional case study below demonstrates how knowing the reasons for your weight struggles can help you to work at resolving them.

> Maria had never thought much about her weight until she was 18. Looking back at her childhood, she would say that she had always been an 'average weight' and never really knew much about dieting. Her parents didn't diet, and as a family they all just enjoyed whatever they wanted to eat. Maria started to gain weight when she started university, which she feels was caused by a combination of stopping the netball training she used to do at college, drinking more alcohol, and eating differently because she was away from home. She ate more ultra-processed foods and had a much lower budget for food shopping. In her mid-twenties, Maria met a partner who liked to

go to the gym and was focused on nutrition, so she joined in with this, lost weight, and felt happy with her body and health for the first time since she was a teenager. She maintained this way of life for many years, also maintaining her weight. Maria regained some weight at 32 when she had her first child, which she put down to craving sugary foods during pregnancy. Her baby struggled with sleep, and Maria was sleep deprived as a result, causing her to continue to eat sugary foods as she felt they would give her energy. Now, at 38, Maria weighs about 4st more than she would like to and continues to eat a lot of sweet foods even though her daughter sleeps well now – she feels that this has become a habit, which she has tried and struggled to break. She also looks forward to 'a treat' at the end of the day, when she gets to sit down with her partner and relax. Exercise has taken a back seat, as she feels that life is just too busy with a school-aged child and a full-time office job. Maria has tried a local slimming club but found it hard to stick to the number of points she was allocated each day.

Looking at Maria's story, she has two times in her life where she gained weight. She naturally resolved her issues on the first occasion, when she met her partner, because his approach encouraged her to eat well and exercise, which she had not been doing at university, hence her weight gain. It is clear that her second occurrence of weight gain, since having her daughter, has been caused by an excess of sugary food, poor sleep habits and lack of physical activity. Trying to stick to a diet will not necessarily help to solve these problems for maria. A diet would not address the mindset that makes Maria feel as though she neds to have sugary foods as a treat every evening. A diet would not offer motivation or inspiration, and could feel restrictive after so many years of Maria eating whatever she wanted. Going back to the point on her timeline where she was happy with her weight, she felt supported by her partner, was exercising regularly, and eating food which was nutritious and enjoyable. Rather than trying more diets, if Maria returned to these key elements of healthy living, which she knows worked for her before, she is far more likely to succeed in losing weight and feeling healthier and happier again. If Maria can ensure that she gets enough sleep, this should help her to avoid being attracted to sugary foods as an additional energy boost, and therefore prevent the cause of weight gain which affected her success previously. Positively for Maria, she doesn't need to follow complicated diets which are hard to stick to – a balanced lifestyle with plenty of tasty, wholesome foods and regular fun fitness works for her, and feels great too. She feels happy that she is working on a permanent solution to her weight struggles so that she can break the cycle and help her daughter to grow up with a healthy attitude towards food and self-care, and with all the tools she needs to keep herself healthy in the long-term.

Maria had two occurrences of weight gain, both with very different causes and triggers. She was able to look back at actions she had taken previously and choose those that had worked well for her. Once you are aware of the root cause(s) of your current weight gain, the next step is to think about the actions you need to take to overcome this. Consider things which have helped you in the past, but remember to question why you were not able to maintain the weight loss on that occasion. If an approach was successful but difficult to maintain, this is not something to return to.

Now that you are aware of the reasons for your weight struggles, you are more empowered to be able to move forward knowing that you are taking aligned and appropriate actions to help your individual circumstances, rather than using a 'one size fits all' approach which may end up making your health and weight issues worse. The good news is that knowing how the timeline of your past has impacted you, you can use what you learn in this book to positively influence what your future timeline might look like, the person you would like to become, and what you would like to achieve over the coming years.

Strategy Summary:

- To know what actions you would be best taking to help you to lose weight, you first need to know how and why you gained weight in the first place.
- Trying to tackle your weight without knowing why you gained the weight could affect your health negatively or could be unsuccessful and frustrating.
- Your weight gain could be caused by a number of different factors, including what you eat and drink, lack of movement, stress, poor sleep, medication, hormones, and genetics.
- Finding your root cause can help to empower you as you live your healthy lifestyle, and positively affect your future health and happiness.

STRATEGY 4: DON'T SET WEIGHT LOSS GOALS.

"Health is a journey, not a destination" (Unknown)

Before we even begin to start thinking about how to lose weight and improve your health, you need to know *what* you want to achieve. Getting into a car and starting to drive with no idea of where you are heading would be a pointless activity, and so would reading this book without knowing what you would like to achieve by doing so. However, I am going to suggest something that you likely won't be used to; don't set weight loss goals! I wrote a great little section on goals – I even developed my own version of the SMART goal-setting process, which you may be familiar with, discussing how setting the right goals for you in the first instance would greatly improve your chances of succeeding with them. I realised that everything I had written would apply fantastically to an area of life like buying a house, getting a new job, or going travelling – a goal with a definite end outcome – but it just didn't sit right with me when applied to weight loss and health, which I see as a lifelong journey rather than a one-time destination. Wanting this book to reflect my true, intuitive beliefs around health and wellbeing, I just knew that I would be pushing the wrong approach if I included my section on goal setting as I had first written it. You need to know what you want, but this needs to be emotional, rather than numerical. I know this because I've been there. Since becoming interested in health and fitness in my early 20s and losing the little bit of extra weight I wanted to lose, my body naturally seems to feel happy at around 65kg.

Being a driven person who believes there is always a way to improve, I was always keen to lose just a few more kg. Now in my thirties, I am far more enthusiastic about feeling good every day, enjoying activities and experiences, feeling strong, keeping my ulcerative colitis and other illnesses at bay, sleeping well, and modelling healthy behaviours for my son. Whatever I do, however I eat, however I choose to live; these are the outcomes I am most keen to achieve, regardless of my weight.

Goals like mine are continual and everlasting. This isn't to say that you shouldn't have goals with an end point, for example, being fit enough to run a 10k or losing enough weight to feel comfortable wearing a bikini. With this kind of goal though, we must be wary of 'arrival fallacy'. Arrival fallacy, a concept coined by Dr Tal Ben-Shahar, in the belief that reaching a certain goal will bring you long lasting happiness, forgetting that it is important to enjoy life right now and to find contentment in the *process* of striving for a goal. The process of working towards a goal is thought to provide as much, if not more pleasure than the achievement of the end result. Studies have shown that excitement is at its highest when planning a holiday as opposed to actually being on the trip! I recently listened to a self-development masterclass by a fabulous coach called Melanie Ann Layer. She told the story of her time spent in Hawaii and her desire to go on a world-famous road trip she had heard about called 'The Road to Hana'. All she could think about was getting to Hana, but the tour stopped so many times along the way to see beautiful sights, breathtaking views, and incredible waterfalls. Melanie spoke about how she enjoyed the sights but couldn't help but worry that they wouldn't have any time left to spend once they finally reached Hana if they continued to stop. Upon reaching Hana, she was surprised to find just a few fruit and trinket stalls, and realised that the magic of the trip was in the journey, not the destination! If you have ever succeeded in losing weight before you may remember how good it felt to achieve consistent losses. How proud you felt when you achieved. How much better you felt as you noticed your body getting smaller, and your health improving. When you reach the weight that you feel comfortable at, you'll then be working at maintaining that weight, which can also be a great feeling, but may not give you the same 'buzz' or feeling of achievement as you got from losing a pound or two each week. Are you hanging all your happiness on the moment you finally reach your goal weight? Are you forgetting to enjoy the process of being healthy and working towards the outcomes you desire? If this sounds like you, remember that if you *were* to arrive at your ideal weight, you would then need to maintain that weight if you are to continue to be as happy as you expected this achievement to make you. And, if the journey to get you there and keep you there makes you miserable, causes stress, or is difficult to be consistent with, you won't feel happy anyway. "It's not a dream body if it's a nightmare to maintain!". If the arrival fallacy alone isn't enough to convince you that you don't need to set a numerical weight loss goal, the following information may contribute to the creation of a mindset in which you focus on how you are feeling consistently rather than what you want to achieve 'in the end'.

Having a numerical weight loss goal is similar to calorie counting, in that the focus is based around numbers rather than feelings. Having a specific number-based weight loss goal can cause frustration and disappointment, as you may work hard, lose weight, and feel much better, but still never reach the initial weight loss target you set for yourself. There are several reasons why this might be the case. You may be looking back to a time in your life where you felt happy with your weight and be aiming to reach that same weight again. However, your body changes over time for many reasons – hormonal fluctuations, pregnancy, and age are just a few. You may find it difficult to reach or sustain that weight again, yet it is possible to achieve the same feelings of contentment at a different weight if you release the attachment you have to that specific numerical goal and focus instead on how you want to feel. If you take part in exercise – particularly resistance training – to support your health and weight loss journey, your body composition will likely be different, with lean muscle tissue weighing more than fat, but improving your body shape. This should be celebrated, rather than seen as a negative! You've likely seen comparison photos on social media of two people who weigh the same but look very different in terms of how athletic, lean, or healthy they appear. This is down to body composition and proves that weight isn't directly related to appearance or how you feel.

Specific weight loss goals may be easy to measure – jumping on the scales tells us straight away whether we are getting closer – but they are not an assessment of how healthy you are, how nutritious your food intake is, or how you *feel* about your health and weight. I'd advise either avoiding the scales altogether or weighing yourself very infrequently. I generally don't weigh myself, and don't keep scales at home, but the gym I go has a set which I jump on a couple of times a year, more out of curiosity or the need to know my weight when filling out a health-related form, rather than a need to see a certain number. It is easy to become obsessed with the number on the scales, and to feel upset when it isn't what you had hoped it would be.

Setting numerical goals may not be the best way to strive for improvements in our weight, fitness, health, and wellbeing, but we *do* need to know what we want in order to be able to work towards achieving it. It is more useful to decided in detail how you want to feel, and other outcomes you would like to achieve or experience, rather than what you would like to weigh. For example, feeling full of energy and doing regular exercise that you love, noticing an improvement in your skin health and digestion, being comfortable in clothes you enjoy wearing, and feeling confident undressing in front of your partner. With these outcomes, they do not rely on reaching a specific weight, and depend on a range of factors including mindset, health, nutrition, and self-care. Of course, weight *does* play a part in how you feel, and 'losing weight' can still be very much a part of your ideal outcome, but I don't feel that there is a need to aim for a specific number of pounds lost or an exact ideal weight. Similarly, setting other numerical or rigid goals, such as drinking 2 litres of water every day or running 3 times a week, may also be unproductive and counterintuitive – although it very much depends on your individual traits and what your motivators are. There may be days where you are less active and the weather is cooler, and you feel the need to drink less water, just as you may want to replace a schedule run with a yoga session at home if it is raining heavily or you are feeling achy and stiff from your last workout. Leaving diet culture behind and working with a mindset focused approach to health also calls for moving away from setting yourself up for failure, ticking boxes for the sake of ticking them, and setting SMART goals just because you have always been taught that they are the best way to get you to where you want to be.

Task:

Journal around the following questions:

1. **How do you feel at your current weight and in your present state of health?**
2. **Before you started to read this book, did you have a weight loss goal in mind? What was it?**
3. **Why did you set this goal for yourself? Was this a weight you previously felt content with?**
4. **Visualise your future. How do you want to be, look, and feel?**
5. **What health and wellness outcomes would you like to achieve?**
6. **Are these outcomes dependant on reaching that SPECIFIC weight?**

When you think about the results you would like from your endeavour to lose weight and become healthier, it is important to ensure that these results match up with the effort you are prepared to put in. To achieve certain outcomes, you will be required to put in more effort than you would need to put in to achieve others. Are you happy to limit your expectation to be able to make life easier for yourself? Or do you want to commit to taking more time for your health and working a bit harder so that you can achieve optimal results? Put simply, if you are not reaching your desired health and weight outcomes, you may either need to reduce your expectations of what you can achieve with your current level of input, or put in more effort to look and feel the way you really want to. Either choice is absolutely fine – this is your journey and your life.

Strategy Summary:
- Don't set number-based weight loss goals – health is a lifelong journey, not a one-off achievement.
- Think about the outcomes you'd like and the way you want to feel each day.
- Be mindful of 'arrival fallacy', where you believe that the achievement of your ideal weight will bring you everlasting happiness.
- Enjoy the journey. Remember 'it's not a dream body if it's a nightmare to maintain'.
- Don't aim to 'get back' to a certain weight that felt good before. This may not be realistic due to changes in your age, hormones, body composition and lifestyle. Do be aware though of where your weight naturally settles.
- Avoid rigid goals in other areas of health and lifestyle too, for example drinking a set amount of water or sleeping for at least 8 hours every night.

STRATEGY 5: FIND INTRINSIC MOTIVATION TO BE HEALTHY.

"You can look for external sources of motivation and that can catalyse a change, but it won't sustain one. It has to be from an internal desire" (Jillian Michaels)

By definition, motivation is simply the reason(s) for acting or behaving in a certain way. In reality, though, it is much more complex than that! Knowing more about motivation and what motivates you could prove to be a game changer as you work on improving your health and losing weight.

Why am I able to say 'no' to a plate of biscuits offered to me when someone makes a cup of tea? Why do I bypass what feels like 90% of the food and drink in the supermarket when I do my food shopping, and only pick out the foods I know are whole or minimally processed? Why do I consistently plan and eat nutritious meals containing healthy ingredients? Why do I go to bed early almost every night? In contrast, why do I get up early to go to a spin class some Monday mornings but not on others? Why did I use a Couch to 5k running app consistently until I achieved the 5k, and then stopped running?!

'Motivation' is a word I've used regularly during my decade in the health and fitness industry. Only recently though have I started to think about motivation at a deeper level, and how complicated it is when considered in relation to weight loss and a healthy lifestyle. I find myself watching people who appear 'motivated' to regularly exercise, to eat nutritious food, and to take good care of their own wellbeing, and noting what their motivators are. I've had conversations with many people to find out what motivates them to commit to the habits they repeat persistently to achieve results. I've read books and listened to podcasts to try to understand more. The concept of motivation is starting to fascinate me!

Well-known motivational speaker Mel Robbins claims that 'motivation is garbage!'. She says that motivation to do a particular thing is either there, or it is not. When motivation is present, it makes it easy to do that thing, but when you are not motivated, it can be very hard to get started. This is why she suggests creating your own motivation rather than expecting it to just show up – and I agree. While there are many theories on motivation, I believe that motivation requires a combination of intrinsic factors (natural, inbuilt) and extrinsic elements (coming from outside oneself), as well as short-term and long-term motivators. While extrinsic motivation can light the fire and help to encourage the acquisition of healthy habits, for long-term, sustainable coherence to these new habits, you'll almost certainly need to look inwards, and consider what really makes you want to change.

The people around you contribute considerably to your extrinsic motivation. A friend can encourage you to go out on a run with them, or they could persuade you to join them for a fast-food feast. I recommend having at least one accountability buddy when it comes to health and fitness. This is someone who will encourage and motivate you when you struggle to find intrinsic motivation – and you will do the same for them, of course. Throughout my journey over the last eighteen years, I have had several accountability buddies, whether they have been aware of it at the time or not, all of whom have helped motivate me to keep going and to enjoy being fit and healthy. I first started to attend fitness classes in my early twenties, and I made a good group of friends there. Knowing that I would see them at a class and that we would get together for a coffee and a chat afterwards offered me a great deal of encouragement and initiated consistency with my attendance. Eventually though, the motivation to get up and go to class became intrinsic, and I would want to go because of how the exercise made me feel. This was just as well really, as when I moved to a new area and started attending a different gym, I was on my own again. Even now, after all these years of being a part of the health and fitness world, I still make use of extrinsic motivation, even though I have good stores of intrinsic motivation available within me too. I love to go to the gym for resistance workouts, but tend to be inconsistent with cardio. I have a local friend who feels the opposite way, so we support each other. She encourages me to book in for spin classes, and I make sure to motivate her to come with me to the weightlifting ones. Sharing transport to the gym helps, as you are more likely to show up when someone else is relying on you. This is all well and good, but if you are reliant on external motivation alone, somewhere along the line there are good chances that you will slip up. When the external source of motivation is temporarily or permanently missing, you may struggle to remain motivated and consistent. I am still much more likely to skip that Monday morning spin class if my friend is not going too!

Luckily, for the most part, I have high levels of intrinsic motivation, and I am able to engage in positive habits and a healthy lifestyle for the sole purpose of wanting to feel good When discussing motivation, I really like the analogy of paying children to do chores around the home. If you offer to give a child money to help with the vacuuming, washing the dishes and tidying up, they are likely to only want to help because they receive the financial reward. If at any point in the future you expect them to help without the lure of money in return, there isn't going to be a very high chance of them being interested in doing so. On the contrary, if you create a culture of pride and respect within the home and talk to your children about how nice it is to have a clean and tidy house, it may take some time, but eventually they are more likely to help without expecting anything in return. The motivation in this case is intrinsic – they want to help so that they can have a nice environment to spend time in. If a child is paid to do chores, one day when they live on their own as an adult and the payments stop, it could be very difficult for them to become motivated to do the housework, as no extrinsic reward is offered.

So, how do you find intrinsic motivation for exercise, eating well and living a healthy lifestyle? Well, a great starting point is to define your reasons for wanting to do those things in the first place. Without a strong enough 'why', it is very likely that you will find it hard to motivate yourself to succeed. A person who is trying to lose weight to be able to qualify for fertility treatment is probably going to be more motivated than someone who is going along to a slimming club just because their friend wants to go.

My own reasons for being motivated are two-fold – firstly, I want to feel as good as I can every single day. I want to be full of energy, look strong and feel healthy. Knowing what it feels like to be constantly tired and to have painful, time-consuming health issues, I much prefer the alternative! Longer term, I look to the future and know that I want to be mobile, active, and physically capable for as long as possible, and to be around to enjoy my son, my loved ones and everything that life has to offer. I know that for this to happen, I need to commit to consistent healthy habits now. Almost all of the time, these two reasons are enough to motivate me. You might be thinking how fortunate I am to be motivated so easily. It hasn't always been this way though, and it has taken plenty of mindset work and self-development to reach this stage. In fact, I have to do this work every day! I remind myself of my values, the identity I want to embody, and the reasons why I want to live the way I do. To achieve this for yourself, it's time to dig deeper into your most important reasons for wanting to achieve weight loss and better health. What is the *most* compelling reason of all for you to lose weight and become healthier? Something so strong that it feels as though you will succeed *no matter what* with this important reason pushing you forwards.

At this point I feel called to say again that weight loss is not something that has to feature among your desires! I am sure that some people set out on a journey to achieve it, or include it in their goals lists or new year's resolutions either because of societal pressures or because they struggle to come up with any other goals which would suit them better. It is okay to be happy with your weight, whatever that weight is. Actually, erase that. It is *desirable, positive,* and *wonderful* to be happy with your weight and your body! Even if you *do* weigh more than you would like to, or aren't as healthy as you could be, if you are not completely compelled to put the time and effort in to change right now, you will be setting yourself up to fail from the beginning. So, if you *are* in that position, and have purchased this book and decided to lose weight for reasons that don't feel aligned, I want you to consider passing the book on to someone who could benefit from it, and go and enjoy your fabulous self – just as you are! In addition, you don't have to want to become healthier – although I highly recommend that you do! If it just isn't something that you are enthusiastic about or motivated by, there is no law to say that you must be healthy!

If you really do want to lose weight and become healthier, let's think about your reasons and locking in your 'why'. We need to ensure that your 'why' is strong enough to carry you through the times where it may seem easier to just give up. Without a really good reason for doing something, it can be difficult to stay motivated, and very easy to just stop altogether, perhaps even fooling yourself into believing that the weight loss and improved health was never meant for you in the first place. What is more likely is that your desire to lose weight is not in alignment with your 'why', therefore causing a sense of disconnect with the outcome and a weaker desire to achieve it. So many people striving for weight loss are doing it in a way that doesn't fit with their lifestyle, personality, and beliefs, and as a result they are not having success.

What is the first thing that comes into your head when you think of your 'why'? Does losing weight and becoming healthier mean more years to spend with your family? Will being slimmer mean that you will feel more confident in yourself? Are you keen to lose weight for your wedding or a holiday? Do you want to be a good role model for your children? Often, people will say that their 'why' is related to their loved ones, or living a longer, better quality of life. "I want to be able to run around with my kids" or "I want to live long enough to meet my great grandchildren". But, funnily enough, although these seem like powerful reasons that would inspire you and motivate you to want to lose weight and be your healthiest self, it doesn't always work this way. If it did, and these reasons were compelling enough, those individuals would have achieved their goals long before now.

I've had some incredibly interesting conversations with my coaching clients about what encourages them, what lights them up, and how these things are often different to what they state their 'why' to be. One lady came to me having had joint replacement surgery a few years ago, and recently found out that her cholesterol and blood pressure were high. She had signed up for coaching under the premise that she wanted to get these readings back within a healthy range. However, a few sessions in, she told me that having an affair years ago prompted her to get into 'the best shape she'd ever been in', whereas wanting to keep her new hips healthy and bring her blood pressure and cholesterol readings down wasn't necessarily proving to be quite as motivating for her! Now, of course I'm not suggesting that being unfaithful in your relationship is the way to kickstart your weight loss, but we can certainly learn a thing or two from this example about how our minds work when it comes to getting motivated to achieve our goals. The reality is that everyone will be motivated by different things, and it's going to be important for you to find out when really gets you fired up to make a start, commit, be consistent and start to achieve. The lady I just mentioned is obviously not hugely motivated by improving her mobility or by preventing any further health problems as she ages. She *was* motivated by excitement, and the things going on in the here and now. How could she illicit those feelings for herself again in ways other than being unfaithful to her partner? Perhaps by travelling to a new country, learning a new skill, taking up a hobby, engaging in an activity which feels risky or exciting, or meeting new friends. By finding something that would bring her similar novelty and excitement, my client might feel motivated enough to lose weight again and become healthier. Her joint health, blood pressure and cholesterol would likely improve, too.

While I find it easy to be motivated by thoughts of the future, others need to know that their hard work will benefit them sooner rather than later. Seeing quick results can act as additional motivation to continue. Knowing *what* you are likely to be motivated by can unlock great potential in your weight loss and health journey. These motivators will be very individual and unique to you, and may feel small, insignificant, niche or even strange! I like to look and feel good, but I am particularly motivated by feeling good about my body when I lay down in bed at night. This is when I would really notice if I was feeling bloated or in pain – something I was used to experiencing most nights when my ulcerative colitis wasn't controlled. I am also motivated by having glowing skin – not from an image conscious perspective, but from a place of knowing that healthy skin means I am eating well, sleeping well, and drinking enough water. I like to wear shorts to work and to the gym, almost all year round. I like that my legs look strong, and this acts as another motivation, especially when it comes to exercise. What are your unique motivators?

Task:

Journal around the following questions:

1. **List some extrinsic motivators that you could use to help in your quest for weight loss and improved health.**
2. **List some intrinsic motivators which could help you to succeed.**
3. **List as many reasons as you can think of**

for wanting to lose weight and become healthier.
4. What is that *one* captivating, compelling reason for wanting to lose weight and become healthier?
5. What *would* happen if you achieved weight loss and better health?
6. What *would not* happen if you achieved weight loss and better health?
7. What *would* happen if you did not achieve weight loss and better health?
8. What *would not* happen if you did not achieve weight loss and better health?
9. Do you feel as though you have identified your true 'why'?
10. Is it enough to push you to succeed? If not, reconsider your 'why' until you have something which feels as though it is.

Strategy Summary:

- Motivation is your reason for doing something.
- Intrinsic motivation comes from within, whereas extrinsic motivation comes from outside sources like friends, family, medical professionals, media etc.
- Having a variety of extrinsic and intrinsic motivators can be very useful.
- Discovering your 'why' can help you to succeed with weight loss.
- Your 'why' needs to be strong enough to compel you to keep going when it feels hard to do so.

PHASE 2: NOURISH AND RELEASE

STRATEGY 6: SWITCH TO WHOLE FOODS.

"Real food doesn't have ingredients. Real food is ingredients". (Jamie Oliver)

So much of the work we do in this book is mindset related, but of course, the actual food you eat plays a huge part too! Probably the simplest and most impactful piece of advice I can give you is to make the switch to a predominantly whole food diet. This means eating foods which are as close to their natural state as possible, rather than those which are ultra-processed. But, what exactly is an ultra-processed food anyway? And why should we be avoiding them? My fellow nutrition students and I had this exact conversation a few months ago during a public health nutrition lecture, when a student asked for the definition of an ultra-processed food. An interesting discussion ensued, but no one definition was decided upon! After doing some more research, a whole range of explanations of ultra-processed foods came to light, including:

- Foods made with ingredients you might not find in your kitchen cupboards
- Foods high in salt, fat and sugar
- Products made of industrially produced ingredients and created through industrial processes
- Foods which have been through multiple processes and contain many added ingredients
- Foods you would struggle to recreate in your kitchen at home
- Foods which are heavily altered from their

natural state
- Packaged foods made by food companies using manufactured ingredients

Ultra-processed foods include things like ready meals, breakfast cereals, cakes, pastries, sauces, sweets, fizzy drinks, crisps, processed meats, and desserts. In contrast, whole foods include meat, fish, eggs, fruits, vegetables, wholegrains, beans, pulses, herbs and spices.

Task: Think about the foods you eat most often. Write a list of them – consider your breakfast foods, lunches, evening meals, snacks and foods you consume outside of the house. How many of these are 'whole foods'?

When we prepare healthy meals or snacks, we are just combining, or cooking with, whole foods. This could be as simple as popping some raspberries and dark chocolate in a bowl for a snack, or pairing vegetables with meat and stock to make a stew. The problem is that in recent years, people are not consuming as many whole foods, in favour of snacks and meals which have already been prepared for them. Processed foods are not the enemy here – ultra processed foods are. Slicing an apple, freezing peas, roasting and grinding coffee beans are all examples of processes which foods undergo, and none of these are harmful to your health. The problem comes when foods are industrially processed and/or made with ingredients which are not whole foods.

Ultra-processed food is a relatively new concept within h
ealth and medicine, and as such, the extent of the effects of consumption are not wholly known.

However, it is thought that ultra-processed foods can cause or contribute to the following:

- Obesity
- Health conditions like heart disease, diabetes and cancer
- Digestive health complaints
- Nutrient deficiency
- Mental health issues like depression and anxiety

On the flip side, whole foods offer the following benefits:

- Better weight management
- Reduction in illness
- Improved immune system
- Better digestive health and more varied gut microbiome
- Increased energy levels
- Improved mood
- Better quality sleep

Task: Take your list of foods from the last task. For any ultra-processed foods, write down replacement whole foods which you could use or

try out instead.

As with everything I suggest, this should not be an 'all or nothing' approach. This is about making changes you can be consistent with, that suit your lifestyle, not about being super strict and then 'falling off the wagon' – remember, this isn't a diet! Our bodies are pretty amazing, and can handle small amounts of ultra-processed food, but we just weren't designed to eat them for every meal.

Strategy Summary:

- Choose whole foods over ultra-processed foods wherever possible.
- Don't feel as though you need to be really strict – this is about what you eat most of the time, not about occasional consumption of ultra-processed foods.

STRATEGY 7: LEARN ABOUT ANCESTRAL EATING.

"Ancestral eating is about connecting with yourself through flavours; it's an act of caring for your body". (Don Marin)

When was the last time you ate organ meat, drank bone broth, or consumed something that had been fermented? In modern society we are missing out on a great deal of powerful nutrition because we have stopped eating the foods that are meant for us, and have shifted towards foods which do not adequately nourish our bodies and minds. Ancestral eating encourages us to avoid alcohol, excess fibre, refined sugar and grains, seed oils, ultra-processed foods, and even cultivated fruit and vegetables that would not have been available before the agricultural revolution, as it is thought that these contain 'plant toxins' which can have a detrimental impact on health. Instead it suggests focusing on eating good quality animal products, healthy fats, fruits, vegetables and fermented foods. I am still learning about this concept, and as with any ideas within health and nutrition, I would recommend doing some reading and research and acting on what resonates with you. I definitely think that there are many elements of ancestral eating that we could benefit from incorporating into our lives, but as always, I would approach this with balance and awareness in mind – I'd never suggest being so strict that you couldn't ever enjoy 'modern' fruits and vegetables, or ingredients that our ancestors wouldn't have had access to!

I particularly agree with the belief that human beings need to consume animal products and plenty of good fats. From my own experience of healing my ulcerative colitis, I know first-hand that eating this way can have dramatic transformational effects on your body, mind and health, but also it makes sense from a nutritional, scientific perspective. Animal products contain protein that is far more bioavailable than plant-based sources, which means it is more easily accessed and used by the body. They also contain omega 3 fatty acids, amino acids, and nutrients like heme iron and vitamin B12, which can be challenging to obtain from a plant-based diet. Animal foods are nutrient dense, which means they contain high amounts of vitamins and minerals in small quantities of food.

One of the benefits of eating ancestrally is the improvement or elimination of health conditions caused by inflammation. This is said to be down to the removal of ultra-processed foods, refined sugar, grains and alcohol from the diet, as these are thought to cause inflammation within the body.

Strategy Summary:
- Ancestral eating is about eating more of the foods that early humans would have consumed, and avoiding more modern, ultra-processed foods.
- Ancestral eating is an interesting concept, which I'd encourage you to learn more about.
- Don't be too strict with ancestral eating – take what resonates and works for you, if anything, and leave the rest.

STRATEGY 8: REFRAME THE IDEA OF TREATS.

"From childhood, we're brainwashed into thinking that junk food is a treat. We're given candy for being good; there's cake and chocolate on our birthday; we go to fast food restaurants on special occasions. The message is clear: this food is special". (Allen Carr)

One of the most important changes I think that you can make in terms of weight loss and management is reframing the idea of treats. What is a 'treat'? Why do you need or deserve 'treats'? Are they *really* 'treats'?

Task:

Without overthinking, list all of the foods that come to mind when you think of the word 'treat'. Answer the following questions with the list in mind:

1. What do you notice about these foods? Is there a common theme among the foods you have listed?

2. When and why do you allow yourself to have treats? How often? What behaviours do you feel deserve a treat?

3. How do you feel when you are consuming treats?

4. How do you feel afterwards?

5. Do you feel that the 'treats' you eat have had a negative impact on your health and weight?

6. Do you think that by having the treats you are really 'treating' yourself?

7. Are there foods that are not on your

list that you would enjoy just as much, and would not cause you negative side effects?

I bet that most of your list is made up of foods that are ultra-processed and high in sugar. Foods like sweets, chocolates, ice cream, cake, and fast food. The difficulty we face is that ultra-processed foods like these are deliberately designed by manufacturers to be appealing, palatable, easy to eat, and addictive! Many companies producing ultra-processed foods employ scientists to work out how to make their products even more desirable to the consumer, meaning that they are almost impossible to resist. The more you eat, the more you want! We are also led to believe by companies and those around us that these foods are good rewards for working hard, or an ideal way to cheer ourselves up if we feel sad, down, or lonely. How many times do you hear the phrase 'oh go on, treat yourself!'?! As a society, we are indoctrinated with the idea from a very young age that sugary, sweet, processed foods are 'treats'. We give young children sweets as a treat, or take them out for milkshakes, hot chocolates, cookies, and cakes as 'a treat'. Have you ever specifically 'treated' yourself or your kids with a healthy balanced meal? Have you ever visited a farm shop and picked out some good quality meat and vegetables as a weekend treat for yourself and your family? It's more likely that you have taken your children to the sweet shop on a Friday after school or rewarded them for an achievement with a trip to a fast-food restaurant. Think about the reality of this. If I am going to treat myself, I want that treat to make me feel good, both in the short term and long term. Eating junk food may provide a quick pick-me-up and a release of dopamine (the pleasure hormone), but the feeling is over very quickly, and long term you are likely to be left feeling guilty and suffering from the effects of eating such foods. You may feel low in energy, notice a change in your skin, have brain fog, or experience digestive discomfort. If you regularly eat these kinds of foods, your health could be at risk – an outcome which does not seem like a treat to me.

Since qualifying as a personal trainer in 2012, I have eaten a healthy, balanced diet, with an occasional ultra-processed offering, which even I believed to be a treat! More recently, I have spent a lot of time diving more deeply into nutrition and learning about the effects of ultra-processed foods on the body, as well as the psychology behind health and weight loss. I'm also far more aware of how different foods affect me as an individual. While researching for this book, I happened to listen to the audiobook version of Allen Carr's Easy Way to Quit Emotional Eating. The book was the monthly pick for an online self-development book club that I participate in, and I almost chose not to listen that month, because I didn't feel that I needed any help with emotional eating. In the end, I decided that I *would* listen to the book with the intention of expanding my knowledge and to learn new ways to help my clients, but I was amazed at how it changed my own mindset too! Now, I could definitely find a lot of criticism with this book, and there were some statements and claims made that I completely do not agree with, including Carr's opinion on certain foods and how unhealthy they are for you. I still believe in balance, and advocate eating what feels right for you. His stance is very 'all or nothing', which I don't think is healthy. Cutting out all ultra-processed foods forever is unsustainable, unnecessary, and extreme. However, since listening, I have removed most ultra-processed foods from my diet and feel *naturally* compelled to avoid them. This is not something I deliberately set out to do, and it hasn't felt hard. Something about the book altered an element of my mindset and reframed how I see 'treats' without me even needing to try to make a change. If I ever do eat anything ultra-processed these days, I am reminded why I usually choose not to! I will either suffer from tummy pain, bloating, a headache, or brain fog, and feel that it would have been more of a treat to avoid the food!

I don't think that it is harmful to the human body to eat ultra-processed foods or 'treats' every now and then, but if the side effects of these foods are not desirable, you have to make the decision whether it is actually worth consuming these foods at all. I recently had a Chinese takeaway with friends. I hardly ever eat takeaway food – mostly because I think it is expensive and I prefer homecooked food. Having said that, I have always found Chinese food to be appealing and tempting and have enjoyed eating it on occasion. About an hour after eating the meal, I started to notice pain in my tummy and began to feel bloated. A few hours later, when I was at home and it was time to go to bed, I found it hard to get to sleep and noticed that my heart was racing. When I woke in the morning I had a headache, and although the bloating had subsided the pain in my tummy lasted for 3 more days! Was this the 'treat' that it was meant to be? I considered this and felt that on this occasion it was not. On the contrary, a week later, my family and I visited a friend with a homemade cheesecake for his birthday. The cheesecake was made with Biscoff spread, which has ingredients I would not choose to eat regularly, including 'candy sugar syrup', palm oil and rapeseed oil. The other ingredients were digestive biscuits, full fat cream cheese, butter, and double cream, so overall the end product didn't feel too 'ultra-processed'! We all had a slice, which I thoroughly enjoyed, and felt no unwanted side effects, so I felt good about the choice to eat the cheesecake, and would choose to eat it again in the same situation. However, the temptation to refer to the cheesecake as a 'treat' is still prevalent! The homemade meal I had eaten before the cheesecake was also delicious and felt like a treat. Ultimately, I want *all* of my food to feel like it is a treat, not just the things that society leads us to believe are treats. That may sound unachievable, or like hard work, but this has really worked for me. Making sure that all of my meals are delicious, satisfying, nutritious, and enjoyable means that I don't feel the need to follow them up with 'sweet treats' or ultra-processed food. This doesn't have to involve lots of complicated or labour-intensive recipes or cooking methods – a piece of homemade bread, toasted and spread with local butter is easy to prepare and makes a really enjoyable breakfast with a good coffee, while a piece of grass-fed steak, sweet potatoes, mushrooms, and broccoli come together quickly and easily to make a tasty evening meal.

Writing about this strategy has got me thinking about life in general, and how, as a society, we feel the need to 'treat' ourselves. This implies that either we have overworked or had a negative experience in order to require or deserve a treat. Moving away from discussing health and weight loss for a moment, what if we looked at life a little differently? What if we tried to live in such a way where we didn't feel the need to counteract the 'bad' parts of our life with food, drink, substances, purchases, or things that are somehow intended to make us feel better? I'm not big on social media trends, but I have heard about the concept of 'romanticising your life', and I really love the idea! It's something I have unknowingly practised for a while, but deliberately try to do it more often now that I know it's 'a thing'. The term refers to enjoying the little things, taking your time, making everyday acts and routines feel special, feeling gratitude, and finding joy within yourself and your life. Examples of romanticising your life could include placing candles on the dinner table, writing a letter to a friend, buying yourself flowers, taking time to enjoy a leisurely breakfast or cup of coffee, making your bed, buying nice cleaning products that you enjoy using, and having a skincare routine. I love the idea of romanticising your life, because all too often we focus only on striving for big future goals, or in contrast, we get stuck in a rut of working, coming home, flopping on the sofa in front of the TV, and repeating daily. By focusing on these little changes, we can make every day feel amazing, even the tasks we may think are mundane or of no consequence. I recently purchased some cushions and extra pillows for my bed, and I feel genuinely happy when I make the bed every morning, plumping up the pillows and making my room look nice. My morning coffee is not just a drink, but a ritual, and I love my evening routine, getting into bed early, feeling fresh from a shower, and reading a book while drinking a cup of herbal tea. I link this practise to the idea that 'how we do one thing is how we do everything'. This concept is the reason why successful, healthy, happy people often approach all areas of their lives in a similar way and have consistent habits across the board. The little things matter! Get up when the alarm goes off, make your bed, have a shower, dress for the day you *want* to have, eat well, keep your house clean and tidy, take time for yourself, your partner, and your kids, and just see how different that feels. Those who are romanticising their lives are taking care in how they prepare food, making their bed every morning, sitting at the table for dinner instead of in front of the TV. They are mindful in how they are living and benefiting as a result. I feel that I approach my life with an attitude of striving towards being my best self in all areas, but also with importance placed on balance and following my intuition. So, for example, I go to the gym regularly, usually on set days of the week, but if I am particularly tired or aching from a previous workout, I am okay with choosing not to go. I work hard within my business but also like to take days off in the school holidays to spend with my son. I value cleanliness, organisation, happiness, and achievement in all areas of my life. I stand up for what I believe in, and live life based on my most important values.

Going back to food, if you can change your mindset from one of 'eating healthy and then having a treat', to 'eating tasty, nutritious food most of the time', I promise that this will make a big difference to how much you enjoy food, but also to your health and chances of losing weight. So many people I have worked with in the past have ended up stuck in a routine of eating 'healthily' during the week and then binging or having 'treat days' at the weekend. I hate the 'cheat day' or 'treat day' mentality! With this mindset, you are still putting the ultra-processed, sweet foods on a pedestal, believing that they are the foods you enjoy the most. Find a tempting, balanced, nutritious recipe, go and buy the ingredients you need, and set aside time to make it. Enjoy making it, present it well, and make mealtimes an occasion. Sit down with your family if you can and enjoy serving them food that you have cooked. Eat as much as you feel you need, but take care not to eat until you are too full. This whole process will feel so good that you won't crave anything else, and you won't feel the need to reach for a 'treat' later on. We are aiming for balance and consistency rather than a situation where your nutrition swings between the extremes of being 'really good' and then 'treating yourself' to counteract that. Sweet foods and snacks are part of a healthy, balanced diet – but try to make them yourself, and seek out recipes which are nutritious as well as satisfying. For example, a homemade banana loaf with nuts, raisins and dark chocolate is a much better choice than a shop-bought cake. If you fancy ice cream, read the ingredients lists and choose one with fewer added ingredients.

There will be times where you want to eat a certain food, but eat it just because you want it, not because you need to treat yourself.

Task:

Journal around the intention of romanticising your life. Write about ways that you already do this and ideas you could start to implement.

Think about the concept of 'how you do one thing is how you do everything'. Do you believe this about yourself? How would you describe the way you currently approach your life and the different elements within it? How would you like this to change?

Strategy Summary:

- We are led to believe that ultra-processed food, fast food, and sweets are 'treats'. This is a belief that most people learn as very young children.
- Food companies deliberately design ultra-processed foods to be moreish and addictive.
- Many people tackle weight loss by going on a diet, depriving themselves of the food they enjoy, then 'falling off the wagon' and binging on treats because they are not satisfied.
- If a 'treat' causes you negative side effects or makes you feel rubbish, it's not a treat!
- Making sure that most of your food is delicious and satisfying moves you away from thinking of food as being either 'health food' or 'treat food'.
- Romanticising your life can help with your mindset around treats.
- 'How you do one thing is how you do everything' – the way you approach one area of your life is likely to be how you approach the rest. Consider how you show up in life, and what you could change to give you a better chance of success.

STRATEGY 9: EAT, LIVE, AND CONSUME INFORMATION INTUITIVELY.

"Intuitive eating means learning to honour your mind, body, and health". (Unknown).

Intuitive eating—a term you have probably heard, but do you know what it means?

Intuitive eating is trusting your inner wisdom to make choices around food that feel good and right for you without influence from diet culture.

The reaction a lot of people have to this concept when they are used to dieting is that they would not be able to trust themselves to eat intuitively. That they would not be able to trust themselves to *not* be on a diet. That their eating would somehow get out of control or that they would not be able to make healthy choices. It saddens me that some people may never experience a sense of freedom around food, where they can trust in themselves to make the right choices for them and their bodies in any given moment and feel at peace with what they have chosen to consume.

Using your intuition is a big part of my approach to health and weight management. You will need to see intuition as you would a muscle – I believe it is something which needs to be trained consistently to get stronger. I am fifteen years into my food, nutrition, and health journey, and I have spent this whole time honing my intuition and learning how to eat intuitively so that I can experience freedom around food. Something which is worth mentioning is that there is no end point to my journey, and there will be no end point to yours. Things will change along the way, but you will need to consider your food and nutrition *forever* so that you can maintain good health and a weight that you are happy with. Learning to eat intuitively enables you to make changes to your lifestyle and eating habits as you move through life, doing what feels good and what suits you at the time. There is a myriad of books and resources out there for you to delve as deeply as you want to into the principles, benefits, and practicalities of intuitive eating, but the following information will give you an introduction and encourage you to begin to move away from diet mentality and towards that of a healthy lifestyle.

Intuitive eating is a term that was coined in 1995, in Evelyn Tribole and Elyse Resch's book 'Intuitive Eating: A Revolutionary Program That Works.' Their ten principles are a great way to learn more about intuitive eating, so do read the book or visit their website if you feel called to. The principles include honouring your hunger, respecting your body, and not succumbing to diets. If you have been caught up in diet culture for a long time, this can all sound a bit daunting. If it helps, write out the list of principles – either from Tribole and Resch's book or from their website - and keep it with you so that you can refer to them regularly, reminding yourself of how to act intuitively around your body and food. Having said that, you do not have to follow intuitive eating as a programme – you can simply take what resonates with you and use it as you see fit, leaving the rest. As with other concepts, methods and ideas, intuitive eating won't suit everyone. Because intuitive eating encourages you to accept your body as it currently is, attempting to lose weight can feel in conflict with this, so this part in particular may not feel aligned if you are embarking on a weight loss journey. Something which those new to intuitive eating may struggle with is the temptation to binge on previously 'forbidden' foods. I feel that intuitive eating needs to be combined with other techniques, such as the identity strategy I share in this book, and reducing intake of ultra-processed foods in order to be successful for weight loss.

Most articles and books you will come across about intuitive eating focus on being mindful about what you eat, how much you eat, and when you eat it. I also want you to extend your intuition to where you get your information from, and how you react to the advice, suggestions, and recommendations presented to you. The media is saturated with health, wellness, and weight loss information these days, and it is almost impossible to decide what to believe, who to listen to, and where to even begin! As I suggest later on in Strategy 16, do what feels *truly* right for you, not others, when it comes to how and what you eat, and how you live your life. It is *so* easy to get swayed by social media, books, and news articles, which lead you to believe you should be eating in a certain way or following new wellness trends. In reality, you are either following an individual who is raving about something that has worked really well for *them*, or a company or organisation wanting to sell their product or achieve an ulterior motive. Fasting, ketogenic diets, going plant-based, drinking smoothies or juices, taking certain supplements, giving up dairy or gluten are all examples of dietary changes made by others that you may be tempted to emulate. When something works well for someone, and it has a big impact on their health or other element of their life, they will talk passionately about it. Reading or listening to accounts of how fantastic it is to have no digestive discomfort after ditching dairy products, or dropping several dress sizes by becoming vegan can make it really tempting to try and do the same, in the hope that you will also experience those results. However, everyone is different, and what works for one person and their lifestyle, personality, and preferences, may be a disaster for another!

When you read or hear health and weight loss suggestions, take note of your first reaction, consider how you truly feel about what is being promoted, and think about how making this change could work for you, including whether it is something you could sustain. Last year I read a book called Fibre Fuelled by Dr Will Bulsiewicz, a leading gut health doctor. It was an interesting book, from which my biggest takeaway was that the health of the gut microbiota relies heavily on having a varied intake of nutrients from as many different sources as possible. I devoured the book quickly, feeling enlightened and excited to put my newfound knowledge into practice. When I reached the meal plan section of the book however, it became apparent that the recipes were incredibly restrictive to me, all plant-based, and after just 3 days I felt hungry, a lack of energy and had cravings for foods which were more appealing, sustaining, and tasty than those suggested in the book. Continuing the plan would have made me miserable! Other people may have felt completely differently, both when reading the book and when following the recommendations, and this is why it is so important to use your intuition when learning about health, food, and weight loss, and only follow what feels really good for you. Keep reading, listening, and researching, and take what you need from each book, article, or podcast. After reading Fibre Fuelled, I have increased my usage of beans and lentils in my meals, and I have also started to add a wider variety of seeds and nuts to my food. So, although the meal plan didn't suit me – unsurprising given how I feel about diets – I was able to make use of a lot of the information contained within the book. More recently, I have been listening to the books written by Davinia Taylor. Again, not all of her recommendations suit me – with my current lifestyle, fasting until lunchtime just doesn't work for me, and if I took all of the supplements she recommended, I'd be spending more on pills and powders than I do on food! I have seen benefits though from some of her suggestions, including taking MCT oil daily, which has helped me to feel more energised and improved my mental clarity, and using an acupuncture mat before bed to aid relaxation and sleep. I also now start my day with a glass of warm water with lemon and a pinch of Celtic salt, which rehydrates me after sleeping and seems to be having a positive effect on my digestion and skin health. Intuitively, Davinia's recommendations and her stance on health and food sit well with me, and I like her honesty and enthusiasm for learning. While she experiments a lot with nutrition and lifestyle, just like I do, her overarching recommendations are to limit UPFs, eat a diet high in fat, supplement where necessary, and utilise different ways of feeling your best and improving your health. If you spend any time at all reading about nutrition on social media you will be bombarded with posts about how oats spike your glucose levels, oats lower your cholesterol, vegetables contain harmful lectins, plant-based diets are best for humans and the planet, carnivore diets heal a multitude of health conditions, and so many more bold claims which contradict eachother. Many of these claims can hold some truth for some people, in certain situations, but are often taken out of context, and can cause the reader to make radical and unnecessary changes to the way that they eat. Ultimately, you have to trust what feels right for you, both in general and in any given moment. I had a sickness bug for the first time in my life last year, and after not eating for about a day and a half, all I wanted was gummy sweets! Perhaps my body craved the healing properties of the gelatine they were made of, or maybe I just needed something fruity and easy to digest. I could have denied my cravings, opting for something which made more logical sense and was 'healthier', but by allowing myself to have exactly what I wanted, I felt better quickly. I have been in similar situations with my ulcerative colitis – prior to a flare up I will crave plain, carbohydrate laden foods, which are 'not very nutritious' in my head, but my body knows that they are easy to digest, and that energy can be quickly released from them. Again, I have to listen, despite what my head is telling me! Continuing to eat the fibre-filled vegetables, beans and pulses that I want to eat will just cause me pain and suffering. I'm not saying that all of this is easy, because it isn't. Even recently I have felt full after my evening meal but have still chosen to have a second helping or more food later in the evening, just because the food on offer was so delicious! I am really mindful these days about how much I dislike the feeling of being too full, and almost all of the time I am able to think about this and stop when I am adequately satisfied. But, as with most of the other strategies I have shared in this book, intuitive eating is a practise – something you have to keep working at, always aiming for 'the best you can' rather than trying to be perfect. Listening to your intuition around food, lifestyle changes, movement, and the information you consume will help you to move away from diet-culture, and towards deciding for yourself what is best for your body and your health. Over time, as you become more used to respecting your intuition, you will be able to develop a better, more enjoyable relationship with food and with your mind and body.

Task:

Journal around what feels true and right for you when it comes to food and lifestyle.

Write about any times you can think of where you have either listened to your intuition about food, or ignored it. How did it feel to honour your intuition or to go against it?

List some social media accounts, professionals, authors, and people you know in real life who you trust and feel intuitively drawn towards in the health and nutrition space.

List those who you feel called to avoid, and consider why.

Strategy Summary:

- Intuitive eating is a concept first written about in 1995 by a dietician and a nutritional therapist. It is based on a collection of 10 principles encouraging you to avoid diets and trust yourself where food is concerned.
- Intuitive eating could be seen as the opposite to dieting. It offers freedom and no judgement, whereas dieting is restrictive and causes reliance.
- Intuitive eating involves eating when you are hungry, eating the amount you need to feel nicely full, enjoying food, respecting your body, and finding forms of movement you like to take part in.
- It is important to be intuitive about the information you are consuming too, as there is an abundance of confusing, conflicting, inaccurate, and sometimes dangerous information out there, especially on social media.
- Always go back to what feels good for you.
- Trust what feels right in the moment. If you are craving something, it may be what your body needs.

STRATEGY 10: EAT TO FEEL GOOD, LIVE TO FEEL GOOD.

"Your diet is a bank account. Good food choices are investments" Bethenny Frankel.

This strategy is one I've recently turned into a bit of a life motto. It came about partly because I needed a simple way to remind my son about how to choose what to eat and how his habits would affect how he felt. I also needed that reminder for myself! I am becoming increasingly aware of how differently I eat and live compared to most of the people I know, and it would be easy to question sometimes whether this is the 'right' approach, and whether I need to put as much energy and effort into my food choices as I currently do. I always come back to my 'why'…wanting to feel as good as possible every single day, and wanting to be healthy and active for as long as possible. The idea of eating and living to feel good becomes a strategy of its own, in addition to finding what works for you. Will this food make me feel good? If it is likely to cause bloating, brain fog, or any other negative side effects then the answer is 'no'! Will drinking alcohol make me feel good? For me, the answer is always 'no', and I made the decision on 1st January 2024 that alcohol was a substance that no longer serves me in the life that I want to live and for the person that I want to be. A hangover is never worth it for me. Does staying up late make me feel good? No, it doesn't - ever! But on the odd occasion, the thing I'm staying up for *is* worth it, so I do make that decision every now and then.

We are all so completely different as individuals, and as such, we all need to eat and live differently to feel at our best. Become a researcher and discover the foods and behaviours that make you feel good, and those that don't. You are now building on the journal task given to you in the last strategy, where you wrote about negative side effects from the food you ate. Continuing with your journal, be mindful of any health conditions, physical signs, mental health symptoms, neurodivergences, sensitivities and intolerances you have, and consider how food and lifestyle habits affect these. This is something I have become much more interested in recently, and while I will always advise against dieting, I do advocate for tailoring your eating habits to help you feel your best. This may involve making changes, cutting back on or removing certain foods, or choosing to eat in a different way. As I mentioned earlier, I have ulcerative colitis, which I control with nutrition and lifestyle as opposed to medication. I have noticed that my symptoms are worse when I eat a lot of vegetables, so I am careful to eat an appropriate amount. I have recently been exploring how I feel when reducing my intake of wheat and other grains, despite previously rejecting the idea that these may cause me issues, probably because I didn't want to go down the route of avoiding them! Moving away from diet mentality and towards the intention of doing what is best for your body is a game changer! If you are lucky enough not to suffer from any health problems or have any unwanted symptoms, simply keep eating the foods that make you feel good!

Task:

List any health problems, conditions, illnesses, mental health concerns, and neurodivergent symptoms that bother you currently.

Become a researcher! Look for books, social media accounts, podcasts, websites, articles, even documentaries on the issues you are dealing with. Make sure these are from reliable, unbiased sources. Find out what you could be doing to help yourself to eat and live in ways that could help you to feel better.

Strategy summary:

• We are all different – our bodies, our minds, our lifestyles and our preferences.

• We need to remember that what works for one person may not feel good to us.

• Start to be more aware of how you feel when you eat certain foods – both physically and mentally.

• Eat more of the foods that make you feel good, and less of those that don't.

PHASE 3: REWIRE AND REBUILD

STRATEGY 11: WORK ON YOUR MINDSET ABOVE ALL ELSE.

"Weight loss doesn't begin in the gym with a dumbbell; it starts in your head with a decision". (Toni Sorensen)

There are so many weight loss resources available to tell you *what* to do, and many even explain *why* you should do those things. For example, 'increase your fibre intake to feel fuller for longer' and 'eat enough good fats so that your body can store and use vitamins effectively'. What is lacking though, in many methods, is the bit that tells you *how* you are going to put those recommendations in to practice consistently when you feel unmotivated, don't what you want, and don't know where to begin. The missing piece of the jigsaw is the mindset work – a piece I feel is just as important as the food you eat and the amount of movement you are doing. In my opinion, mindset could be the most important part of your quest to lose weight and keep it off. With The Honest Weigh, you are working on changing the way you think in order to make the physical changes easier and more sustainable in the long term. Most diets only consider the food that is being consumed, and perhaps the amount and type of movement you are doing. In this strategy, we are going to focus on the underlying psychology and mindset underpinning your weight and health status, and how altering these things can prompt you to make different choices and change elements of your lifestyle. In turn, this will have a knock-on effect on what you eat, the way you live, and how you managed your weight.

I am a *huge* fan of self-development. Learning

about self-development and committing to practising it regularly has changed my life – and that isn't an exaggeration! Self-development is the deliberate and continual pursuit of improving your skills, knowledge, and qualities in a variety of areas. A commonly used tool in the world of coaching is the 'wheel of life'. Completing a wheel of life can provide insight into the elements of your life that you feel least content with, and therefore would benefit from working on. Because I take a holistic view on health and weight, I think the wheel of life is a valuable tool to encourage you to think about how other areas of your life can affect your health and weight, and how your health and weight could be affecting those areas.

Task:

Complete the wheel of life. Assess each area and give it a score out of 10, with 10 being as happy as you could possibly be in that area, and 1 being completely unhappy. Colour each segment up to the corresponding number. Answer the following questions:

1. **What are the two lowest scoring segments of your wheel?**
2. **Write down one or two small actions that you could take that would help you towards increasing the scores attached to these two areas of your life.**
3. **Would improving your lowest two**

scoring segments help you to lose weight and become healthier? If so, how?
4. How does your health and weight currently affect the two lowest scoring areas of your life?
5. Would improving your health and losing weight have an impact on the score you chose for those segments?

The wheel of life is a working document that you can repeat periodically to see how your scores have changed and how self-development is helping you to improve the different areas of your life.

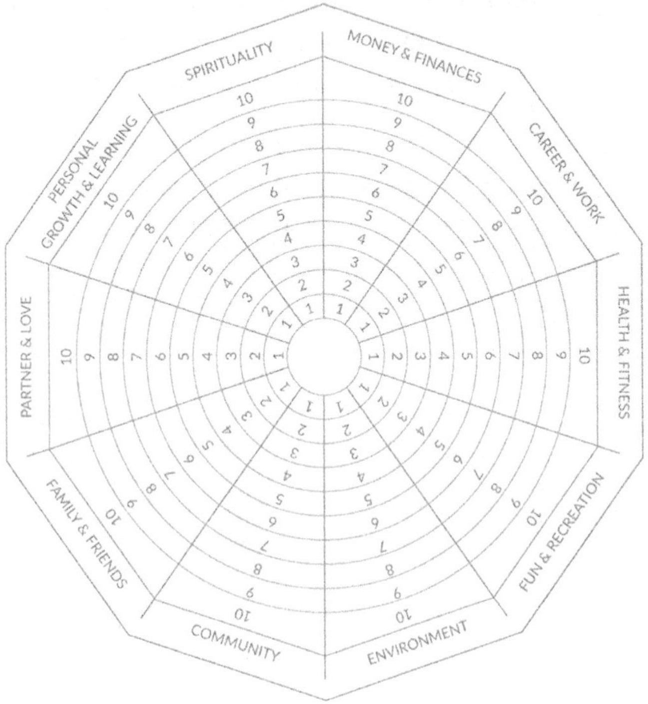

I truly believe that the answer to most of our health and weight related problems can be found by combining self-development with balanced nutrition, feel-good movement, and a lifestyle which respects your body and mind. Does this seem achievable to you right now? Your answer to this question may depend on your mindset type, so we will take a look at that before we go any further. Psychologist Carol Dweck's theory describes two types of mindset – the fixed mindset and the growth mindset. She believes that the type of mindset we have plays an essential part in what we think we can achieve, what we desire for ourselves, and the life that we live.

Fixed Mindset Traits	Growth Mindset Traits
Believes that intelligence is set in stone and cannot be changed	Believes that intelligence can be developed
Avoids and dislikes challenges	Embraces and seeks out challenges
Gives up easily	Shows tenacity in the face of setbacks
Dislikes and does not utilise constructive criticism	Asks for feedback and takes on board suggestions for improvement
Resists putting in effort	Knows that effort will result in positive outcomes

Acts negatively when others succeed	Gets inspired by the success of others

Task:

Using the mindset table, assess your own mindset and decide whether you currently have a fixed mindset or a growth mindset. If you think that you have a growth mindset, you can move on from this task and continue reading – you are already set to do really well with the rest of this book! If you think that your mindset is fixed; don't panic! Working on each point in the mindset table, consider what you could do to help switch your mindset from fixed to growth. Write one or two simple actions for each point, and start to implement these immediately. Copy the table on to a piece of paper and place it somewhere you will see it often. Think about how your daily actions contribute towards your mindset type and try to ensure that the actions you take are helping to work on developing a growth mindset.

One of my favourite ways of improving your mindset is by using gratitude for your current situation. Depending on your experience of working with gratitude to date, you may already be on board with this, or you may wonder how being grateful could possibly help you with your health and weight! In a challenging or troubling situation, you cannot always control what happens, but you do have some control over how you react. By being grateful for the good that can be found in a situation, even when the overall circumstances are less than desirable, you are focused on the positive rather than the negative, and this can help you to feel more hopeful that you will get the outcome you want.

Task:

Start a gratitude journal. Every day, write down between 5 and 10 things that you are grateful for, and the reason why. For example, 'I am grateful for the water that is supplied to my home, as I am able to bathe in it, cook with it, and use it for washing my dishes and clothes' or 'I am grateful for my boss because she allowed me to take Thursday afternoon off so that I could watch my son's school play'. Try to write down different things each day. See how the power of gratitude builds as you continue with this practice.

Write a specific gratitude list for your weight and health. The fact that you are reading this book suggests that you want to change your weight and health, but try to focus on the positives within this area, for example 'I am grateful that I live in a beautiful area where there are some lovely places to go for walks', 'I am grateful that my partner is happy to support my lifestyle changes', or 'I am grateful that I have been inspired to improve my health now and not later

in life'. Spend around 20 minutes on this list, writing as many points as you can think of, and read it back to yourself daily.

Founder of Ford Motor Company, Henry Ford, famously said "Whether you think you can, or think you can't, you're right". This alludes to the idea that a growth mindset can hugely contribute towards outcomes, achievements and successes. Of course, he is not suggesting that simply thinking of the outcome you want will bring it immediately into reality. What he was implying was that you first must have the *belief* that something is possible. (even if you think it may take a lot of hard work or many attempts before there is a chance that it can actually happen). There are people across the world who have achieved the most amazing feats, all starting with the planting of a seed of belief that the end result *could* be possible for them. The film 'NYAD' documents this point fantastically, sharing the true-life story of swimmer Diana Nyad, who swam from Cuba to Florida, a distance of 110 miles, without resting, aged 64. This had never previously been achieved by anybody, but Diana *believed* that she would be able to complete the swim, despite everyone around her thinking she was completely delusional! It took her five attempts. You can apply the power of belief to your health and weight loss. You have the ability to decide that you will succeed. In fact, you *must* believe that it is possible.

Think about the language you use when talking to others and to yourself. Over the years I have worked in the health and fitness industry, I have heard *so* many women say things like "I know I'll never be a size 10, but I'd be happy to just lose a few pounds", "I'm so weak, I gave in and had sweets at the weekend", or "It's alright for her, she's always been thin". These are examples of thoughts coming from a fixed mindset. One way of counteracting these negative thoughts and words are affirmations. Affirmations are positive statements or mantras which you can use to help you change or enhance your thoughts or behaviour. Repeating affirmations can help you to instil belief in yourself and challenge negative self-talk, gradually changing the way that you think about yourself and your potential.

Task:

Create a set of affirmations that you can use to strengthen your growth mindset and instil the self-belief you need to become healthier and happier, and to reach a weight you feel comfortable with.

Tips for writing and using your affirmations:

- **Keep it short and sweet – aim for an affirmation which is easy to remember and repeat. This will increase the chances of it being useful to you.**
- **Use language that feels true to you – if 'I look and feel awesome every**

day' feels more natural to you than 'I am manifesting my healthiest, most attractive self', go with the words that suit you and your personality best.

- Be realistic – the affirmation must feel comfortable and as though it could be true for you, where you are right now, while also being expansive and encouraging of growth. "I am building trust in myself that I am capable of living a healthy lifestyle" may feel more honest and effective for you than "I am the healthiest person I know".

- Turn negatives into positives – if there is something you struggle to do or haven't been able to achieve, write an affirmation which says that you *can*. I often used to say, "I'm just not a runner" but when I started to tell myself "I am getting better at running every time I try", I was able to improve my ability and feel happy that I was taking part in this healthy habit. This has also worked incredibly well for me with punctuality, organisation, and getting up early. I am now 'a morning person who likes to get up at 6am', and 'I like to be organised as it makes life so much easier!'.

- Write in the present tense – "I *enjoy* choosing healthy foods as they make me feel energised and vibrant" works better than "I *will* choose healthy foods so that I can feel energised and vibrant". The latter phrase frames this as a choice you will make in the future, rather than something you are working on right now.

Interact with your affirmations often. Try 'habit stacking', as recommended by James Clear in Atomic Habits. This involves adding your new habit (the affirmations) to an existing habit which is already well established. For example, repeating your affirmations after you clean your teeth. You may also find it helpful to display one of your affirmations as your laptop or mobile phone screensavers. You could even try setting an alarm on your phone with your affirmation attached so that you are automatically reminded of it regularly.

Strategy Summary:

- Diets don't usually consider mindset, and often focus only on food and fitness.
- Working on your mindset can help you to change your lifestyle, lose weight, and become consistently healthier.
- The wheel of life shows how different areas of your life could be affecting your weight and your health, and vice versa.
- The best way for most people to tackle their weight and improve their health is with a combination of nutrition, mindset work, movement, and lifestyle changes.
- If you do not already have a growth mindset, working to develop one will help you to achieve the health and weight loss outcomes you are keen to see.
- Gratitude can help you with your mindset in general and is a fantastic activity to engage with daily. It can also be powerful in helping you to feel more positive and less overwhelmed with the changes you want to make and the weight you would like to lose.
- Affirmations are a great reminder of your potential, abilities, and possibilities.

STRATEGY 12: CONSIDER THE PERSON YOU WANT TO BECOME.

"The only person you are destined to become is the one you decide to be". (Ralph Waldo Emerson).

Who are you?

Are you happy with the person you have become? The person you are evolving to be? The life you live? The way you feel every day? The way you show up in life?

If you are answering 'no' to these questions, it's time to take a look at how you can make changes so that you *do* feel aligned with your identity and how you live your life.

There is a fantastic chapter in Atomic Habits entitled 'How Your Habits Shape Your Identity (and Vice Versa)'. I'd recommend reading the entire book to gain valuable and insightful support in building new healthy habits and breaking any existing habits that you would rather not keep. Chapter 2, in particular, discusses how we tend to focus on changing our *outcomes* rather than altering our *identity*, and how the latter can be much more effective, especially long term.

> 'Imagine two people resisting a cigarette. When offered a smoke, the first person says "No thanks. I'm trying to quit". It sounds like a reasonable response, but this person still believes they are a smoker who is trying to be something else. They are hoping their behaviour will change while carrying around the same beliefs. The second person declines by saying "No thanks. I'm not a smoker." It's

a small difference, but this statement signals a shift in identity. Smoking was part of their former life, not their current one. They no longer identify as someone who smokes.'

Your identity as a healthy person is what will motivate you to continue to eat well, move your body, take great care of yourself and work on maintaining your weight loss long after you finish reading this book. Like your health and your relationship with food, your identity is something that you will be working on for the rest of your life.

I *love* being a healthy person. I enjoy going to the gym, attending health and wellness events, and talking to likeminded friends about all things health. I find myself choosing to wear fitness clothes when I have no plans to workout, I am one of those rare people who enjoys food shopping, and I like browsing social media for tempting new recipes to try. Spending time in my kitchen preparing delicious food for me and my family to share is time well spent. I love getting up at 6am and knowing that I'm doing something good for myself by meditating, journalling, and eating a healthy breakfast, rather than staying in bed and snoozing the alarm clock like I used to, feeling stressed that the morning wasn't going to plan. I love that my son wants to be healthy too, and that I am setting a great example and being the best role model I can be for him. I feel proud that bringing him up in a healthy household is having noticeable effect on him now, but that it could have a positive impact on him for the rest of his life too. I enjoy paddleboarding and cold water swimming, and it feels great to feel happy with my body when going about these activities. One of the best feelings ever is waking up energised, full of vitality, excited for the day ahead, physically fit, and strong, with clear skin, and a digestive system that is working well. These are the feelings I strive for daily. I have to strive for them, as they are not things which will just occur on their own, but it doesn't feel like a chore to do so. These outcomes are reliant on the actions I take and the way I choose to live. They are reliant on the person I choose to be. My identity is that of a healthy person.

It wasn't always that way though. As a teenager I spent my weekends at the pub with friends, consuming pints of lager and fast food, staying up late, giving little thought to nutrition or health. If I wasn't out on a Friday or Saturday night, I'd be at home eating sweets in front of the TV! Looking back, I feel grateful that I made the decision to make changes to my lifestyle in my early twenties. Fortunately for me, I persevered for long enough to discover a passion for being healthy, and in the end, my identity began to change. Over the last 18 years I have used my identity as a healthy person to keep my weight at a level I have been happy with. This is not something that you do once and continue to reap the benefits from. Rather it is a continual process, which sometimes involves checking in with yourself and making changes to the way you are thinking, behaving, and living. It isn't always plain sailing. Early in the pandemic, in April 2020, I had a realisation which led me to question the person I was becoming. I had not been exercising for several months, allowing work to take over, and using the excuse of being too busy to go to the gym. My eating habits were not as balanced as they usually were, and I'd gained about a stone in weight. The pandemic hit, and with lockdown preventing me from working for several months, I had to face up to the fact that lack of time was no longer stopping me from exercising and eating well. Like most other households, we jumped on the Joe Wicks bandwagon, getting up and religiously joining in with his morning workouts. I have huge respect for the inspiration and motivation that Joe provided for people of all ages and abilities across the country, but the novelty soon wore off for me. Doing squats and burpees in my living room didn't inspire me to keep going, and I didn't notice the kind of changes that I wanted to see in my fitness and body shape. This completely validates my belief that for changes to be sustainable, they must suit you, your lifestyle, and your preferences. These can all change, depending on your age, circumstances, and the stage of life you are in. Just a few weeks into lockdown, we moved to a house in a little village about 10 minutes away from the town we had previously lived in, and it felt like an opportunity for a fresh start with my health and wellbeing. I signed up to the Couch to 5k app, and although running wasn't my usual activity of choice, the challenge of starting from scratch, along with great scenery in my new village made it a lot more enjoyable! I did this in conjunction with Caroline Girvan's EPIC workout series on YouTube, which was based on resistance training. My love of all things fitness and health was being revived, and I realised how much I had missed being THAT person! We decided to turn our spare room into a gym and purchased some equipment from the internet. When it arrived, it felt flimsy and poorly made, and I just knew deep down that the answer was to send it back and join a gym again, so that I could use decent equipment and spend time in a place which would help me to maintain my healthy lifestyle—and maintain the identity of a fit and healthy person. As soon as gyms were open again, I signed up for a leisure club membership at a hotel near my house, and it was the best decision I could have made. I have recently renewed that membership for a third time, and I now cannot imagine a time in my future where I won't belong to a gym or leisure club. Since 2020, I have become even more interested in health and wellness, and particularly nutrition. I spend a lot of my time these days learning more and implementing healthy behaviours in my own life. Being a healthy person really is such a strong element of my identity now. Looking back, I think that if I hadn't addressed my health and fitness at that point and been really honest with myself about why my habits had changed, I'd have said goodbye to that part of me for good, and settled back into a life where wellbeing wasn't a priority. I may have eventually ended up being someone in need of reading this book, rather than the person writing it.

Thinking about the women I have worked with over my time as a health and fitness professional, I can wholeheartedly say that those who have succeeded for the long-term are those who have worked hard to assume the identity of a health person. They have made brave and bold changes to who they are and how they live. They have not dieted but have committed to a healthy lifestyle with no set destination or end point. They were willing to make the changes that were needed to get them the outcomes they wanted to see. I know that I have influenced many of these women, and encouraged them to make changes and feel better about themselves, but the shift in identity in the end *always* came from within themselves. This is the hard part – I can't do this for you!

Have you been using dieting as a way to feel better about yourself? I wonder what would happen if we swapped dieting with self-development? Working on defining and embodying the identity of the person you really want to be. Reading, learning, trying out new routines and ways of thinking instead of restricting what we eat. Exercising in ways we love instead of punishing ourselves to burn the calories we think we overate. Meditating, taking ourselves to bed early, having fun, talking to our friends on a deeper level than just 'what have you been up to?'. Engaging in habits and behaviours which make us feel so good that we naturally *want* to feed ourselves well, with nourishing, balanced food, which in turn contributes to this expanding feeling of wellness. If I were to add up all the time I spend each week on self-development, health, and wellness activities, it would probably equal or surpass the amount of time I spend working. This includes exercise, food preparation, meditation, reading, writing, listening to podcasts and engaging in different ways of learning. It doesn't have to be this way for you though – it is important that your lifestyle suits the identity you want for yourself. I am the healthiest, happiest, and in the best shape I've ever been. Is it a side effect of the self-development or just a coincidence?

Task:

Journal around the following questions:

1. **Who do you want to be? How do you want to show up in the world?**

2. **Let's get visualising, and journalling about *who* exactly this person is. Be as**

detailed as possible, using the following journal prompts.

3. How do you currently spend your day?

4. How do you spend your day as your happiest, healthiest self?

5. What books, tv programmes, music and entertainment do you consume?

6. What books, tv programmes, music and entertainment do you consume as your happiest, healthiest self?

7. What is your social life like?

8. What is your social life like as your happiest, healthiest self?

9. Who are you spending time with currently?

10. Who are you spending time with as your happiest, healthiest self?

11. How do you feel each day?

12. How do you feel each day as your happiest, healthiest self?

From now on, I want you to focus on becoming that person. I recommend that from this moment forward, your identity when it comes to food and weight is that of the person that you want to become. No diet can be as powerful as this. By

GEMMA MULLINGER

focusing on how you would like to feel, the life you wish to live, how you would like to be seen by others, and the habits and characteristics you would like to have, you have already turned your situation around, from focusing on that which you don't want (your excess weight) to that which you do (being your happiest, healthiest self!)

Strategy Summary:

- Your health, weight, and happiness are directly linked to your identity – the person you show up as in the world.
- To make a change for the long-term, your identity must shift.
- Swapping dieting for self-development is a healthy and positive change you can make for excellent results across the board when it comes to your health and happiness.

STRATEGY 13: EXPLORE YOUR VALUES.

"When your behaviour is in line with your values, it is less of a struggle to achieve and maintain change" (Joyce D. Nash).

I can't write about identity without discussing values. I first recognised the importance of core values about 5 years ago, when the topic was broached while I was working in a café with a few friends. We had decided to meet up to work on our businesses together, and before we got to work, Katy, a passionate and dedicated coach, suggested an activity to discover our top core values. This was something I'd never done before, and although the activity was simple, the process and results have been powerful and informative for me ever since, and something I often talk to others about. Discovering my own most important values – freedom, balance, gratitude, purpose, and health – really helped me to curate my life in alignment with the things that are most important to me. Do you know what your core values are? If not, then the next task will help you to discover them. If you already have an idea of the core values which are most important to you, the task will act as a reminder or confirmation of these, or possibly offer you the opportunity to see if these still feel aligned.

Task:

Let's discover your own core values! Read through the list of values below and write down all of those which feel important to you. Add in any values that are important to you that have not been included in the list. When you reach the end, read through your own list, and choose the 20 values which are most important to you. Repeat this process, reading through the list of

20 and reducing it to 10. Finally, choose the most important 3-5 from that list. These are your top core values.

Abundance
Acceptance
Accomplishment
Accountability
Accuracy
Achievement
Adaptability
Adventure
Affection
Alertness
Ambition
Assertiveness
Attentive
Authenticity
Awareness
Balance
Beauty
Boldness
Bravery
Brilliance
Calmness
Capability
Careful
Caring
Certainty
Challenge
Charity

Cleanliness
Clear
Clever
Comfort
Commitment
Communication
Community
Compassion
Competence
Confidence
Connection
Consistency
Contentment
Contribution
Control
Cooperation
Courage
Courtesy
Creativity
Credibility
Curiosity
Decisiveness
Dedication
Dependability
Determination
Devotion
Dignity
Discipline
Diversity
Efficiency
Empathy

Endurance
Energy
Enjoyment
Enthusiasm
Equality
Ethical
Excellence
Excitement
Experience
Expertise
Exploration
Fairness
Faith
Fame
Family
Fearless
Fidelity
Fitness
Focus
Foresight
Forgiveness
Freedom
Friendship
Fun
Generosity
Giving
Goodness
Grace
Gratitude
Growth
Happiness

Hard Work
Harmony
Health
Honesty
Honor
Humility
Humour
Imagination
Independence
Individuality
Inner Harmony
Innovation
Insightful
Inspiring
Integrity
Intelligence
Intuitive
Joy
Justice
Kindness
Knowledge
Lawful
Leadership
Learning
Logic
Love
Loyalty
Mastery
Maturity
Meaning
Moderation

Motivation
Obedience
Openness
Optimism
Order
Organization
Originality
Passion
Patience
Patriotism
Peace
Playfulness
Poise
Positivity
Power
Productivity
Professionalism
Prosperity
Purpose
Quality
Recognition
Respect
Responsibility
Restraint
Results-oriented
Rigor
Security
Self-actualization
Self-development
Self-reliance
Self-respect

Selfless
Sensitivity
Serenity
Service
Sharing
Silence
Simplicity
Sincerity
Skilfulness
Solitude
Speed
Spirituality
Stability
Status
Stewardship
Strength
Structure
Success
Support
Surprise
Sustainability
Teamwork
Temperance
Thankful
Thorough
Thoughtful
Timeliness
Tolerance
Toughness
Traditional
Tranquillity

Transparency
Trustworthy
Understanding
Uniqueness
Unity
Vision
Vitality
Wealth
Welcoming
Winning
Wisdom

Q: Do you feel that you are currently living in alignment with your core values most of the time?

Q: Do your core values feel really true to you?

Q: What could you do to embody each of your chosen values even more within your everyday life?

Q: How could doing this impact your weight, health, and wellbeing in a positive way?

If you find that your values are not linked to health and wellbeing, try to make a connection in some way. For example, if 'adventure' is one of your top core values, being physically fit and healthy can help you to enjoy adventures more, and enable you to take part in more activities and experiences. It may even impact your potential to earn money to pay for those adventures!

Similarly, if 'community' comes out high on your list, being healthy means that you may be able to contribute more to your local community, or be a part of community groups which are centred around a certain activity that you fancy trying, such as walking or swimming. Values are an important part of any mission for behaviour change or new habit formation, and linking your top core values to health can help you to want to focus more on improving your health. If you have been struggling for some time to achieve a particular outcome, such as weight loss, perhaps the outcome you are trying to achieve doesn't align with your values. If you struggle to connect any of your values with your desire to become slimmer, fitter, and healthier, you may need to question that desire, and whether it is strong enough to make it worth continuing to try. Give yourself permission to stop striving for something if it doesn't feel aligned with what you really want. It may be helpful to ask yourself *why* you felt called to strive for that outcome in the first place. Was it because your GP suggested it? Did your partner make a comment about how you look? Are you struggling to fit into certain clothes? Are all your friends going to slimming groups? Or do you feel a real pull towards improving your health for your own sake? Do you really want it that badly? Does it mean *that* much to you? Are you content remaining as you are?

Strategy Summary:

- Knowing what your core values are can help you to develop your identity even further, and encourage you to live in alignment with what is most important to you.
- Focusing on your values can offer you increased motivation to lose weight and live a healthier lifestyle.
- You will probably be able to link health, weight, and happiness to each of your core values in some way, and realise that improving those areas would enable you to embody those values more closely.

STRATEGY 14: MOVEMENT, HORMONES, SLEEP AND STRESS.

"Weight loss is the side effect of living a healthy lifestyle". (Unknown)

In addition to dietary changes, your weight loss and health journey will be supported hugely by other healthy lifestyle habits. In this strategy I want to touch upon four of these – movement, hormones, sleep, and stress. You'll need to do your own additional reading on these areas if you feel that you need more support with them, and you'll find thousands of great books and resources covering different areas of each of them in detail.

Movement is an important part of weight loss and living your healthiest, happiest life. We all know that exercising is good for your body, but I think it is almost as important for your mind as it is for your muscles! For me, exercise is a ritual which releases happy hormones, allows for effective stress relief, adds discipline to my day, and just makes me feel good. I have some of my best thoughts in the gym, and can often be seen scribbling notes in my weight log book, or tapping them into my phone, recording ideas I've had for my business or something I'd like to try. Going to the gym after the school run in the morning is as natural to me as cleaning my teeth. To be able to feel this way about movement, and to successfully incorporate it into your life as a permanent feature, it is important to choose activities that you love and can remain consistent with – whether these are gym sessions, fitness classes, yoga videos on YouTube, walking groups, or even a fun hobby like rollerskating, horseriding, or dancing. It's beneficial to take part in a range of different types of movement regularly, but I recommend that strength training features among these in some way. Strength training is, in my opinion, one of the best things you can do for your body, mind and longevity, and the earlier you can start including it into your exercise schedule, the better. Strength training helps to improve muscle strength, bone density, can help with weight management and has positive implications on mental health and mood. We can start to lose muscle as early as age 30, but the rate of decline increases in our 50s and 60s, and becomes even more significant as we age further. Strength training, along with a nutritious, protein-rich diet can help to mitigate the loss, meaning we are less likely to suffer from muscle weakness, reduced mobility, struggles with everyday activities, and increased likelihood of injuries and falls as we age. Strength training makes up a high percentage of my weekly exercise – I aim for 4-5 gym sessions each week, all of which are wholly resistance based, but even 1 or 2 is enough to make a real difference. There is no shortcut or cheat code when it comes to exercise – you will have to take time out of your day to do it. But there are ways you can make it feel more enjoyable and even more productive if you feel that you are short on time. Try listening to podcasts while you work out, exercise with a friend so that your workout doubles as a social occasion, listen to your favourite music, or exercise outside so that you are also getting fresh air and spending time in nature.

Task:

If you are not already exercising frequently and consistently, write a list of exercise types/ activities that you enjoy doing or would like to try.

Commit to starting one or two of these within the next week. First make the preparations. Do the research if you need to - find a local club, venue, class or session. Dig out your trainers and fitness gear. Ask a friend to join you. Put it in the calendar. Get started!

If I had a pound for every time I've spoken to a woman who asks me what to eat 'to help with the menopause', I'd be incredibly wealthy! Now, I'm not a doctor, I'm not a hormone specialist and I haven't been through the menopause myself yet, so I'll encourage you to seek help and support from a variety of other sources in addition to this book if this resonates with you. Also, we mustn't forget that hormones are not just about the menopause, and they are not just about the sex hormones affecting our monthly cycles. Hormones are chemical messengers which play a variety of roles within the body, including growth, reproduction, energy levels, blood pressure, stress control, sleep, and organ function, and for these to operate optimally we must nourish ourselves well and consider our lifestyle. Again, I'll encourage you to read further around this if it interests you, or if you have questions about a specific area, but I wanted to briefly touch upon some changes you can make to support your hormone health.

Here are my top 10 practical tips:

- Take magnesium – it helps with the production and balancing of hormones, and although it can be found in a wide range of foods, supplementation is a good idea for most people to ensure adequate intake. You may not be aware that there are many different types of magnesium, and each is effective in different ways, and can aid with different issues, for example, magnesium glycinate is great for sleep, and magnesium citrate supports digestion.
- Include more fat in your diet – we have been brainwashed to believe that 'fat makes you fat', but this is not true, and eating a low fat diet can actually be detrimental to our health in many ways. We need fat to be able to produce and regulate hormones, and also to be able to utilise certain vitamins which support the production of hormones. Don't be afraid of consuming more fat – you may be

surprised at how much better you feel for it.

- Cut back on sugar – eating too much sugar affects the way that insulin works in the body, causing fluctuations in blood sugar, which can then lead to a range of heath problems. Also, excess sugar can cause other hormones to be unbalanced, including cortisol, leading to chronic stress, and female sex hormones, exacerbating menopause symptoms.

- Eliminate or reduce alcohol consumption – I gave up alcohol in January 2024, and it has been one of the best choices I have ever made. I feel fabulous for it! Because of this though, I have to be really careful not to let my enthusiasm come across as an insistence that everyone else should also give up drinking too! I'm always happy to chat about my experience of going alcohol-free, but I tell it as it was for me, without making any suggestion that others should do the same. I do, however, recommend cutting back on alcohol, as it can have many serious health consequences, some caused by or worsened by its effect on hormone production and balance.

- Work on your gut health – this is an important one. Did you know that the gut microbiome can influence hormone production and regulation, but also that hormones play a part in your gut health? Yes, it's a two way street! Consider eating more prebiotic rich foods like onions, garlic, apples, asparagus and cocoa, and probiotic rich foods like yoghurt, kefir, kimchi and cheese.

- Practice good sleep hygiene – having recently had a spell of struggling to sleep myself, I feel even more 'qualified' than usual to talk about the importance of sleep! It's another two way street here – not sleeping well enough can cause hormone dysregulation, and having hormonal issues can impact your sleep. It is very common to hear women who are going through the peri-menopause to complain of poor sleep quality. It is really important to implement good routines – going to bed at the same time and getting up at the same time every day, even at weekends! Turning off screens and devices a few hours before bed, allowing your body and mind to relax, perhaps with a hot, caffeine free drink and a book, keeping your bedroom cool, and avoiding overstimulating activities like working or exercising too late. Sleep meditations can be helpful, as can journalling before bed to free your mind of any thoughts that may keep you awake.

- Consciously keep on top of your stress levels – stress can trigger the release of hormones like cortisol and adrenaline, which can then cause digestive problems, weight gain, sleep problems, anxiety, high blood pressure, and other health implications. Try to address the root cause of regular stresses rather than using superficial approaches to temporarily soothe yourself. Consider why you are stressed and what long term solutions you could begin to action.
- Consume enough protein – protein is needed for the production and regulation of many hormones, and also plays a crucial role in appetite and satiety. Ensure you are consuming at least 1g of protein per kg of body weight, by increasing your intake of meat, fish, eggs, good quality full fat dairy products, nuts and seeds.
- Exercise – movement can have a positive and negative influence on hormones, so it's important to get the balance right with this. Exercising too much can cause cortisol surges, which can have a similar effect on the body to excess stress. In general, exercising regularly but sensibly, at an appropriate intensity, can help with the release of mood-boosting hormones, metabolism, reducing stress hormone levels and minimising the effects of

menstrual cycle or menopause hormone fluctuations.
- Relaxation – I struggle with this one myself sometimes! Switching off and allowing yourself to relax is absolutely necessary if your body is to work correctly and efficiently, and for hormone production, regulation and balance. For me, I have to schedule my relaxation daily, as if I didn't, it wouldn't happen! My routine involves a short morning meditation, just after waking, as this helps me to transition into the day in a relaxed and positive state. I also use an acupressure mat every evening before getting into bed for about 15-20 minutes, and I find that this helps me to relax my body and calm my mind ready for sleep. I listen to a sleep meditation as I fall asleep. You need to find what works for you where relaxation is concerned. You may find that stopping at lunch time and spending some time allowing yourself to sit and reflect works better than a guided meditation. Or you may find a walk with no music or conversation works best for you.

This moves us quite nicely into thinking about sleep. In my opinion, getting consistently good quality sleep is more important than anything else you can do for your health. It can have a huge impact on your weight, too. In comparison to exercise or nutrition, for example, sleep is harder to manipulate, and although there are many things you can do to help improve your sleep, ultimately you have less control over it than you do your food intake or exercise output. Despite the fact that you cannot make yourself sleep well, there are plenty of sleep hygiene tools and ideas you can implement, which can really help both physically and psychologically. My first recommendation is to set a wake up time and a bedtime, which you stick to every day, even at weekends. My own sleep improved massively when I started doing this, and as a result, I found that I was more productive, happier, and felt healthier overall. I wake up at 6am and go to bed at 10pm, which gives me a sleep window of 8 hours. Ideally, this would be a bit longer for me, taking into account the time it takes to get to sleep, but now that my son is older and goes to bed a bit later, I find it hard to get settled any earlier, and my early wake up time is important to me, as it allows me an hour before he wakes in the morning to complete my morning routine before the day starts. Do what works for you, and what feels natural – if you are not an early morning person by default, don't feel as though you need to force yourself to get up early – unless your work or other commitments decide this for you! Try to avoid screen time for a few hours before bed. Not only is it thought that blue light from devices can disrupt your ability to sleep well, but also the stimulation provided by the videos, social media or work can also keep your brain active for longer than it needs to be. Instead, try to spend your evenings doing activities that allow your mind and body to relax – good options may include cooking dinner, chatting to loved ones, a gentle walk in nature, spending time in the garden, reading or taking part in a calming hobby like crafting, colouring, art or writing. As mentioned above, a meditation may also be a nice way to wind down before bed. I find that having a 'caffeine cut off point' helps too – mine is lunchtime (around 1pm). I definitely notice that it takes me longer to fall asleep if I've had coffee in the afternoon! Finally, I recommend making sure that your environment is conducive to good sleep. I'm a big fan of a simple bedroom – just the basics with some cosy touches, a comfy bed and good quality bedding. Keep your room tidy and clean. Try a sunrise alarm clock if you struggle with waking up. I got mine about 5 years ago, and I now love it so much I even take it when I go away! When you are refreshed and well rested, your day starts well and you are likely to make more intentional choices when it comes to food and movement, rather than being reactive or impulsive because you are tired. When you are tired, you are far more likely to reach for sugary foods, which you perceive will give you an energy boost, but are actually more likely to cause an energy slump after consuming them.

Task:

Give your sleep routine an audit – consider your current routine, and take note of any actions you could take to improve your sleep. Do you need to set a wake up time and bedtime? Does your environment need a refresh? Can you think of some ways to spend your time in the evenings other than scrolling on your phone or watching TV?

Stress is something that we all have to deal with at some point in our lives, and it comes to us all in different ways, for different reasons and we react differently to it. Stress can impact our body physically, as mentioned previously, and our mental health can be hugely impacted too, having a knock on effect on our lifestyle, daily habits and ultimately, our health. When stress becomes too much to deal with, our food choices ay change, and we are less likely to find time for movement and the rituals and routines that make us feel good. Implementing a calm, effective daily routine that works for you can really help reduce stress day to day, and help you to feel more in control of what is happening. Exercising and eating well, no matter what is happening around you can help you to feel as though you are doing something good for yourself despite feeling stressed, and this can help to create a stronger identity for yourself as someone who is resilient, organised and committed to health and self-care. Even choosing one thing to stick to, no matter what, can act as a positive anchor – for example, meditating first thing in the morning for 10 minutes, or reading a chapter of a book you are enjoying.

Strategy Summary:

• Choose types of movement you really enjoy and can stick at. Think outside the box, and consider fun activities like rollerskating or dancing as well as gym based workouts or classes.
• Incorporate strength training in your routine regularly for best results, both now and as you age.
• Remember that we have many different hormones working within our bodies to enable a variety of bodily functions to occur. Hormonal health is not limited only to the menstrual cycle and the menopause!
• Our hormones work best when we are well fed, well rested and relaxed.
• Sleep is hugely important to our health and weight! We are far more likely to make choices which hinder our success if we have not slept well.
• Consider improvements you could make to your sleep routine in order to have a positive effect on your health and weight loss.
• Stress can also impact our health and weight. Try to work on the cause of any stress rather than utilising quick fixes.

STRATEGY 15: TELL YOUR OWN FOOD LOVE STORY.

"Food brings people together on many different levels. It's nourishment of the soul and body; it's truly love". (Giada de Laurentiis)

Your relationship with food is something which begins when you are a baby and is affected by all manner of influences as you age. From your very first taste of food, you will be subconsciously taking in the actions and reactions of those around you; listening to what they are saying about food, noticing their facial expressions, looking at what they are eating, developing your likes and dislikes, and building up your own unique relationship with food and eating over time. Every single person's story will be different – even siblings can have very different experiences. When trying to discover the root cause for your weight struggles in Strategy 3, you may have found that your upbringing was one of the biggest influences. In fact, I feel so strongly that childhood is one of the most influential factors in your relationship with food that I already know I want to write a second book—one aimed at parents and parents-to-be who have struggled with their weight, with the intention of helping them to intercept this negative cycle before their children can be affected by it too. When children start socialising outside of their immediate family unit, additional influences come into play, including friends, school culture, and eventually, as they grow up, work, media, and romantic partners.

You'll almost certainly have heard the term 'emotional eating', which is often attributed as a contributing factor for weight gain. Correct, when in reference to persistent unhealthy emotional eating habits, but I think we must remember that eating *is* emotional, and we can't and shouldn't want to change that. We could try and take a cold, hard 'food is fuel' stance on eating, but the truth is that food *does* bring pleasure and comfort, and many different emotions are felt when sharing food with others - giving your baby their first solid foods, discovering food from different cultures when on holiday, summer picnics, and eating at birthday celebrations, parties, weddings, and funerals. When you recognise that having a healthy relationship with food can have a whole host of emotional, physical, and social benefits, a new food love story starts to unfold. Here's mine:

> "I love sharing food with my family and friends. I give homemade food as gifts. When I eat out with others, we rarely have our own meals, instead preferring to opt for ordering small plates, sides, and platters for the whole table to share. I really enjoy introducing my eight-year-old to new tastes, meals, and food experiences. I love watching him enjoy his food. I like talking about food. I look forward to food. I adore recipe books. I am a fan of pairing activities or places I love with food —my favourite beach with the gorgeous Sri Lankan curry they serve from a cabin there, paddleboarding followed by a BBQ, or a cup of tea and a slice of homemade banana

loaf with a really good book. I have a real thing for leisurely breakfasts at the weekend, with delicious food, coffee, and interesting conversation. I actually enjoy going food shopping. In the winter, when it's cold and wet outside, I love getting settled in my kitchen with a recipe and all of the ingredients to cook up a feast, with some music playing in the background. In the summer, I like eating outside, and being a bit more spontaneous with what I eat and when. I like having theme nights at home, based on the cuisine from another country, serving up homecooked dishes with all the trimmings. I appreciate it when super simple foods are done really well—toast made from excellent bread, with proper butter, good cheese and biscuits, or high cocoa content dark chocolate. Visiting a farm shop makes an excellent day out for me! I know when I am full and when to stop eating. I feel comfortable saying 'no' to foods I don't fancy or would prefer not to eat. I get a buzz from helping others to learn more about food. Mealtimes are moments where I reflect on my day and chat to my loved ones about theirs. Food is fun, nourishing, therapeutic, and enjoyable. Food is one of my greatest loves".

A diet wouldn't allow me to live out my food love story. It would feel restrictive and remove the joy that I get from food. Food is integral to how we live our lives. It serves so many purposes in addition to simply keeping us alive.

Eating with others is hugely important, and I recently discovered that there is a word to describe the practise of doing so! Commensality is defined as 'the act of eating together'. As someone who loves to share food experiences with friends and family, this has become one of my new favourite words! The reported benefits of commensality are vast – improved mental and physical health, acquisition of good habits, communication skills, and that individuals are more likely to try new foods when eating in the company of others. Personally, I make a point of having as many breakfasts and evening meals with my partner and son every week as possible, and feel grateful every day that the lifestyle I have created allows me to prioritise this. We each discuss the best part of our day, and what we are grateful for, and have done this since my son was two years old. Commensality is helping to shape how we are as a family, and helps us all to have a better relationship with food. It's a part of my life that I am extremely proud of, and I can already tell that I will look back on it fondly when I am much older.

Task:

I want you to explore your relationship with food by writing your own food love story, similar to the one I have shared with you above, including

your own feelings about food, and how it brings you joy.

List ways that you could embrace 'commensality' and improve your mealtime experiences with others, or eat with others more often.

Strategy Summary:

- Everyone has their own unique relationship with food, starting from when they are a baby.
- Your relationship with food is influenced by many factors, including your parents and others around you, your environment, financial factors, the country you live in, and things which happen in your life.
- Your relationship with food is one which is continually changing throughout your life.
- Emotional eating is often seen as a causative factor in unhealthy eating habits and weight gain, but we need to recognise that eating *is* emotional, and serves purposes other than simply physical fuel for our bodies.
- Commensality, or eating with others, is important in creating a great relationship with food, and in being healthy.
- Writing your own food love story can help you to realise how important food is within your life, and how you can enjoy a positive, healthy relationship with food and eating.

PHASE 4: SUSTAIN AND THRIVE

STRATEGY 16: FIND WHAT WORKS FOR YOU.

"The only way you're going to stick with anything long term, be it weight loss or something else, is to tailor it so it works for you." (Shelli Johnson).

Hopefully, by reading thus far, you will have turned your back on the idea of dieting and come to terms with the fact that there is no magic pill to help you lose weight. The truth is, health is very individual, and what works for someone else may not work for you, and following recommendations from others could even be detrimental to your health or your goals. From here, it's about finding out what *does* suit you, and what works to help you to reach your desired outcome within the context of your preferred lifestyle.

Christopher Gardner's DIETFITS study (2013-2016) aimed to discover whether a low fat or a low carbohydrate diet would be more successful in resulting in weight loss and overall positive health outcomes. If I were to make an educated guess on the outcome, I'd say that the low carbohydrate diet would work best. However, the results showed that 'a low-fat diet and a low-carb diet produced similar weight loss and improvements in metabolic health markers. This indicates that you should choose your diet based on personal preferences, health goals, and sustainability' says Gardner. The DIETFITS study shows that even if a particular diet or way of eating makes sense scientifically, it can affect people differently and will not suit everyone, highlighting the importance of doing what works for you as an individual, and what feels good to you.

One thing that we can be sure of, which applies to absolutely *everyone* wanting to lose weight, is that a holistically healthy, balanced lifestyle is imperative to your success. This should be our starting point; always at the centre of everything we do. However, everyone's *version* of a healthy, balanced lifestyle is completely different. The way you approach health and weight loss will vary depending on your lifestyle, dietary requirements, and preferences. It is not a case of a 'one size fits all' approach, which, as mentioned earlier in this book, is where diets often go wrong. When someone writes a diet plan or weight loss book, it is usually informed by and based upon the things that work for them, and the things that they believe to be true. Someone who loves to cook, lives alone, and works part time will come up with a very different meal plan, exercise schedule, and set of recipes than someone who has a busy full-time job, two young children, limited cooking skills and a low budget for food. This is why it is essential that the creator of your healthy, balanced lifestyle is YOU!

I talk a lot to anyone who will engage with me about food and nutrition! I know vegans, vegetarians, carnivores, omnivores, people who are gluten-free, dairy-free, those who fast for extended periods, and those who try to eat as 'cleanly' as possible. They all eat the way they do because that is what suits *them* best, and fits with their beliefs. The man who drives my son's school bus has been following a carnivore diet, and as a result has reversed type 2 diabetes and feels healthier than he ever has before. One of my best friends has recently used a 30-day healthy living protocol, avoiding inflammatory ingredients and ultra-processed foods, and she has improved her sleep and energy levels massively, and will continue with most of the recommendations. Another friend stays away from gluten and dairy indefinitely, feeling that these exacerbate health problems for her. Even my 8-year-old has learnt to notice which foods make him feel good, and which make him feel 'pants', as he describes it! Listening to other people's views on food and nutrition is so interesting to me, and I love reading and learning about the subject. Learning about the effects different foods and ways of eating can have on your body can be helpful, but ultimately, I'd advise eating to feel good. I don't mean eating the foods that *taste* good – although we obviously do want to do that, too! I am talking about listening to your body, and recognising the foods which make us feel vibrant, well, and energised, and knowing which ones make us bloated, give us brain fog, stop us sleeping well, cause our skin to break out, or worsen existing health problems. We are all different, and we must remember this when deciding how to eat. As we move away from dieting, we can move towards individualised eating.

In my work as a weight loss coach, I never offer menu plans these days. Quite frankly, whenever I have given them out in the past, they have been a waste of time! A meal plan is only useful if you have created it yourself, considering your own preferences, budget, cooking skills and foods that you fancy eating at that point in time. I like to eat a different homemade breakfast every day of the week, with options including Bircher muesli, Greek yoghurt and fruit, homemade granola, scrambled eggs, bacon, sourdough toast, smoothies, many varieties of pancakes, smoked salmon, mackerel, avocado, and more. The variety not only helps me to consume a wider diversity of nutrients, but also gives me more enjoyment, prevents boredom, and keeps my young son interested in the food that I am serving up to my family. On the contrary, I have slim, healthy friends who eat the same breakfast every day without fail, and they love it – and they find that it helps them to maintain a healthy weight. They are happy to tuck in to the same thing daily, as it saves them time, effort and money, and forms part of their routine. I know people who swear by batch cooking, and dedicate a day or two each month to cooking up large pots of food and decanting it into containers to stash in the freezer to keep them going over the next few months. Some fill their slow cookers every morning before leaving for work so that food is ready and waiting on their return, and others prefer to cook their meals fresh as they are needed. There is no right or wrong, and that is the beauty of *not* being on a diet. When you follow a diet, you are trying to adhere to someone else's ideal. The fashion equivalent of wearing skinny jeans because everyone else is, when you know that the straight leg variety suit you so much better!

But, where on earth do you start when working out what suits you best? Finding what works for you in terms of food, nutrition, fitness, and wellness really is a case of trial and error! Don't be put off by this. There is so much enjoyment to be found in this process! Try out different ways of eating, experiment with a variety of foods, ingredients, recipes, meals, and menus. Take note of what makes you feel good. Which foods make you feel filled with energy, maintain healthy digestion, give your skin a glow? Which meals get you excited for dinner time? Which combinations fill you up and leave you satisfied? On the flip side, which ones do not?

The concept of individualisation applies to other areas of a healthy lifestyle too – not just food. Getting up early to exercise might really suit some people, whereas others like to get away from their desks at lunchtime for a short session. I was coaching a client recently on exercise and suggested some different options for incorporating strength training into her routine.

She didn't fancy any of my suggestions, and for a few weeks resisted the idea of strength training entirely, because gym and class environments just didn't resonate with her. I stressed the importance of doing something which she enjoyed and felt right, but also that strength training was something that would help her progress and mindset massively. A few weeks later she contacted me to say that she had found an app which offered strength training incorporated with yoga, and that she found it enjoyable and easy to stick to, particularly because she could do it at home while her children were there. Putting it simply, if a recommendation doesn't suit you, you just won't do it consistently, and it won't have the benefits that it is being recommended for. Therefore, it is more productive, and it will feel better if you choose to do things in a way which really works for you.

Fortunately, we have a wealth of resources available to help inform and educate us. I am a self-confessed food, wellness, and nutrition geek! I love to listen to podcasts, talk, and read about the subject. I am open minded, and willing to have my opinions and beliefs challenged, and love to try new things, but always settle on what feels good for *me*. I take what I need from everything I hear and read, and leave the rest. I want you to do the same. Learn. Develop. Try things. Use your intuition. Do what feels truly right. Following this advice will give you better results than any diet ever could, and help you to build the foundations for a healthy life ahead of you – forever. Immerse yourself in information and research, and learn about the nuances of nutrition, health, and fitness where you find it interesting, but please don't stress yourself out with it all.

One problem with taking specific food and diet recommendations, in addition to the fact that they may not suit you, is that this information can become out of date as new research is undertaken. An example of this is coffee. Once thought to be harmful to your health, it is now hailed by some nutritionists and doctors as a 'health food' because of the polyphenols and positive impact on gut flora. Similarly, cheese used to be demonised by many because of its high fat content but is now seen as a good way to make your gut microbiome more diverse. I prefer to make more general recommendations which individuals can work with however they see fit. In terms of nutrition, focus on reducing ultra-processed foods and increasing consumption of whole foods instead. Make it easy for yourself to lose weight and be healthy – don't get distracted by complicated rules and regimes. Feel free to try things out and make changes where they feel good to you, and where they suit your individual health needs. For example, cutting back on foods high in fibre if you have a digestive condition, or reducing oxalate rich foods if they worsen your arthritis.

Task:

The following journalling prompts encourage you to think in more detail about the changes you are willing to make, and non-negotiables for your lifestyle. For example, "I am not prepared to go to the gym but I am prepared to exercise at home" or, "I still want to be able to drink as much alcohol as I want every Friday night, but I am willing to stop drinking fizzy drinks, squash and milkshakes daily".

What are you NOT prepared to do in order to achieve weight loss and better health?

What ARE you prepared to do?

Keep a food diary for a week – not the usual kind, where you list everything you eat! I want you to note down any foods which cause you negative side effects, like those discussed above. If this happens, on each occasion, journal around whether you feel that the food you ate was worth the side effects you experienced. For example, you ate a takeaway and felt bloated afterwards. You would choose to eat it again if you could go back in time, because you enjoyed it so much. Be mindful that the foods that cause you negative side effects may be ones which are hailed as 'health foods', for example kale or nuts.

GEMMA MULLINGER

Strategy Summary:

- If your approach to losing weight and improving your health doesn't make you feel good, you will struggle to stick to it for any length of time.
- It is imperative that any changes you make to your nutrition, exercise, and lifestyle are personal to you.
- Finding what works for you can be a case of trial and error – attempting different ways of eating or exercising and deciding whether it is a good fit.
- Use reputable resources to learn about health and nutrition.
- Keep a track of how foods make you feel – eat more of those which make you feel good and try to avoid those which have any negative side effects.

STRATEGY 17: BE PASSIONATE ABOUT YOUR HEALTH.

"Passion is different from interest. Those who are just interested in things have the 'wish', but passionate people have the 'will'" (Israelmore Ayivor).

I am truly passionate about my health and wellbeing. Are you? When I first started working specifically with women in the fitness industry, I tried to create what I knew my clients and potential clients wanted – an easy way to lose weight without having to commit too much, change too much, pay too much, or alter their way of thinking. For years I worked on this, and for years I was wrong! Of course, what I have just described is impossible! The magic pill these people are looking for doesn't exist! I won't try to pretend that it does. As a qualified and well experienced health and fitness professional, I am not here to tell people what they want to hear. I want to be truthful and try to help others to become healthier and happier for the long term, in an ethical, safe, healthy, and balanced way; *not* to try and create shortcuts or gloss over what it takes to be successful. Think about the people you know who have had success with staying healthy and managing their weight. I can guarantee that they have had to invest time, effort, and maybe money to be able to achieve the results they now enjoy. I want to be completely honest about what I believe is involved in achieving long term success with health and wellbeing, and being able to lose weight and go on to maintain a weight that you are happy with indefinitely. The nutrition and lifestyle advice you will read in this book is simple, but this does not necessarily mean it is easy to commit to.

You know what to do but struggle to do it! The ideas you are reading about in this book may differ from the health and weight loss advice you have received before. I wanted to give you something which will help to prevent you from spending a whole lifetime chasing health, fitness, wellbeing, and weight loss, but never achieving it because you are approaching it in the wrong way. What I suggest instead is spending that lifetime *enjoying* looking after yourself and taking consistent action to be healthy. This is a change of mindset which I believe is essential. You might not like some of the concepts I share, because they quash the dreams that you had of a magic pill or quick fix that allows you to carry on exactly as you are and still drop the pounds. It frustrates and upsets me to see so much unhealthy, dishonest, and misleading information shared about weight loss, and I really want this book to be different from anything else currently available. I had to include a strategy based on passion because that is what created this book. An unwavering passion which has built in layers over the last eighteen years, becoming stronger and more defined, and in the end, impossible to ignore. I've changed my mind about certain ways of doing things, found the industry hard to be a part of, and even walked away for a time. Passion brought me back here. Passion gets things done, gets people fired up to take action and make things happen. Passion is what makes you stick at something even when it is hard, because you believe it is worth it.

Passion is essential for the journey that *you* are currently embarking on. Your body, your health, and your happiness are the most worthy recipients of your passion that I could think of. I truly believe that without passion for your health, your wellbeing, and your life, you will never achieve the results you want – or you will spend your entire lifetime dieting in an attempt to succeed. Whatever your current thoughts are about health, fitness and taking care of yourself, you will need to dig deep and find, reignite, or develop a passion for it.

Task:

Use the following prompts to journal around your current situation and explore the passion you have for your health.

What is the topic that you feel *most* passionate about in your life? This can be absolutely anything – conservation, travel, nature, animals, yoga, crafting, cars, charity, books, parenting, etc.

How do you *know* that you are passionate about this topic?

Do you currently feel as passionate about your health as you do about your chosen topic?

Can you *imagine* feeling this passionate about your health?

What do you think it would take for you to become this passionate about your health?

I almost finished this strategy here, but I realised there was a question which I would need to answer before we could move on. 'How *do* you become passionate about something you do not yet have a passion for?' I hope that the strategies on becoming the person you want to be, and values have gone some way towards helping with this, and I know that the upcoming motivation strategy will support you in creating that passion too. The following advice may also provide some guidance on how to ignite a passion for your health that you may not yet be feeling.

Start by learning more about your body, health, and nutrition. Follow reputable social media accounts about these topics, listen to podcasts, and read books. You won't resonate with everything and everyone, so find resources that feel appealing to you and make you want to read or listen more. As you learn, start to implement different practices, methods, recipes, and recommendations. Make a batch of nutritious homemade granola, follow a yoga workout on YouTube, try a simple morning routine, or download a health and wellness audio book. Do what feels good. Stay committed, keep learning, and keep doing. Start to talk to others about what you are learning and how you feel about it and spend time with people you know who are already passionate about their health. Ask them for their suggestions and support. Most people I know who love health and wellness would be more than happy to offer help and advice to those just starting out on their journey. In fact, the people I know who are passionate about health relish the opportunity to talk about it! Stay consistent and do something each day which makes you feel healthier or improves your knowledge. Just keep going, even when it feels hard!

Strategy Summary:

- Passion for your health is essential. Without it, you will always struggle with consistency and commitment.
- You will be responsible for your body and your health for your whole life. Enjoy taking care of them; don't resent this responsibility.
- Your body, health and life are the best things you could dedicate your time to.
- To become more passionate about your health, start to learn more about it. Follow reputable and appealing social media accounts, read books, and listen to podcasts.
- Talk to others about their passion for health and learn from their experiences.

STRATEGY 18: STEP AWAY FROM PERFECTION.

"It's not a diet. It's not a phase. It's a long-term lifestyle change." (Unknown).

I have alluded to this a few times already, but I think it's worth affirming at this point how absolutely essential it is that you are thinking 'long-term' when undergoing a lifestyle change. I know how tempting short-term fixes are, but I hope that everything you have read so far has helped you to understand why you need to steer clear of them, and *how* you can do this. By giving up diets forever, our aim is to move away from a culture of deprivation and unrealistic pursuit of perfection, and towards a culture of flexibility and consistency. Striking a balance between flexibility and consistency will make it easier to succeed in making sustainable changes that benefit your health and happiness and allow you to enjoy a sense of balance. Rather than swinging between extremes of strict dieting and giving little thought to your health, it is much better for you to practise balance over the long-term.

Flexibility enables you to make changes easily – in the context of health and weight loss, this could mean that you adapt how you eat and exercise through different stages of your life, allow yourself to eat whatever you fancy when you are at a party, or stay at home instead of going to a scheduled workout class if you don't feel like going. It's okay to make changes when you feel they are needed. If the way you eat and live is inflexible, too difficult, and not aligned with your intuition and beliefs, you will struggle to commit in the long term. Life changes, commitments change, and you go through different stages in life, where you will need different things. Becoming a parent may make you feel as though you require a more relaxed routine, but you might also be keen to increase your energy through the food that you eat. As you get older, the amount of food you need might decrease, and your ability to spend lots of time preparing food may change. Being ill can alter the way you exercise and eat, and life changes like divorce and bereavement can also have an effect. It is important to allow yourself flexibility in the way that you eat and live.

Consistency is the reliable repetition of the same, or similar behaviours over time. Things like planning your meals every Sunday, cooking your meals from scratch most nights, going to bed at roughly the same time every night. This doesn't have to mean strict perfection, but I like to think of consistency as 'a commitment to doing the things that help you feel good most of the time'. As I sit writing this strategy, I am enjoying an afternoon of rest at home after a busy work week. I usually go to the gym on a Sunday afternoon, and feel very committed to doing so. However, on this occasion, I felt called to be flexible with my usual plans and allow my body to relax. I can't remember the last time I missed a Sunday workout, so I don't feel that this choice affects my consistency. Flexibility and consistency go hand in hand. It is important to create the right relationship between the two – that is, giving yourself enough freedom and potential to make changes, but also being committed enough and doing what is required to be healthy and happy most of the time. One salad or one gym session will not take you straight away to your ideal weight, just as one piece of cake or missed workout will not cause dramatic weight gain or ill health. It is the way you live day in, day out that will have an accumulative effect on your weight, your health, how you feel, and the results you notice. James Clear writes in Atomic Habits about how 'habits are the compound interest of self-improvement'. Tiny changes seem to make little difference when considered in and of themselves, but when repeated over months and years, the impact on the overall desired outcome can be massive. "If you save a little money now, you're still not a millionaire. If you go to the gym three days in a row, you're still out of shape. If you study Mandarin for an hour tonight, you still haven't learned the language. It's only when looking back two, five, or perhaps ten years later that the value of good habits and the cost of bad ones becomes strikingly apparent".

For consistency to occur, flexibility must also be present. A problem people regularly encounter when dieting is the 'all or nothing' mentality, which causes them to strive for 'perfect' eating and feel a sense of failure when they stray from that path. Have you ever been on a diet, eaten something you felt that you 'shouldn't have had', and then believed that the whole diet was ruined? I bet that you then went on to continue to eat the foods you had been trying to avoid, followed by a realisation at some point in the future that you *do* in fact want to lose weight, and that you would have to 'start all over again'. This cycle is what often stops people from achieving success with diets, and unhelpfully causes them to believe that perfection is the only way to lose weight. Not only is perfection very difficult to achieve, and is not sustainable, but it can also have a seriously negative effect on mental health and your relationship with food and wellness. I want you to let go of the need for your eating habits and lifestyle to be perfect and aim instead be content with the balance that comes from living in a consistent, flexible way.

I was listening recently to a podcast conversation between Steven Bartlett and Bryan Johnson, in which Johnson discussed his blueprint for promoting longevity. This meant taking over 100 medications and supplements each day, eating within a strict calorie allowance, and restricting eating to just a few hours each day, fasting for the remainder. Steven's stance on this was that 'in pursuit of not dying, I don't want to not live', and to me this epitomises why balance is needed in relation to food and lifestyle. Now, of course, *my* balance will be different to *your* balance, Steven's balance, and Bryan's balance. Bryan claimed to have 'never been happier' than since living his life this way. I listened to him talking about his lifestyle and couldn't help but think that it seems excessive, and obsessive, but *he* doesn't feel that way. Some people think that the way I live looks a little bit like too much hard work, but I couldn't imagine being any different now.

For actions or habits to become sustainable and provide you with lasting results, you need to feel good about doing them week in, week out, for a long time to come. Okay, booking a six-week block of Pilates classes is great, and will have a positive effect on your body and mind, but if you don't continue or progress at the end of the six weeks, the results will not be sustainable. Whatever you do, in relation to food, exercise and lifestyle, needs to fit around your existing commitments and appeal to your own likes and preferences. To be able to keep going with the way you eat, move, and live you need to incorporate balance.

Balance not only looks different for different individuals, but also varies from day to day for the same person. There are no hard and fast rules as to what balance means or needs to embody. We want to be heading away from the idea that some behaviours are 'good' and some are 'bad' in respect of your weight, health and fitness, and instead focus on *feeling* good. You shouldn't feel the need to 'offset' every piece of cake or lazy day with a salad or challenging workout – balance isn't transactional. The components and behaviours that make up your lifestyle blend together to create a way of living that feels natural, enjoyable, and truly aligned. Ultimately, if you and your lifestyle are not aligned, you will struggle to achieve the outcomes you desire, or you will be strict on yourself and miserable in your pursuit of your goals.

While you will need to discover your own groove when it comes to flexibility, consistency, sustainability, and balance, I can suggest some ideas that may help you. One habit I highly recommend trying is weekly menu planning. I have been planning my meals a week ahead for about 10 years, and it is a habit I stick to consistently each week, because it truly works for me. Not only does it save time every day, but it also makes my food shopping trips much easier and means that I am more likely to eat diverse and nutritious food. It enables me to be prepared and prevents excess food waste. I sit down every Sunday morning with a coffee to complete my menu for the following week, and I love spending the time searching for tasty food to include. Rather than seeing this as a chore, I have turned it into an enjoyable ritual. I use cookbooks, Pinterest, Instagram, and websites to find recipes to fill my plan, including what we will have for breakfast, lunch, and dinner. You may decide to plan only for your evening meals, only for weekdays, or to choose the meals you will eat but not assign them to the days of the week, deciding on the day which ones you want to have. Make the process your own and give it a try! If menu planning suits you it will feel like something you will *want* to continue with. If not, it isn't imperative to carry on.

It may also be helpful to try planning in advance your exercise and physical activity. This will very much depend on how busy you are, and how motivated you are to exercise. Writing a gym session, walk, swim, yoga session, or fitness class in your diary may help you to be more consistent. I use Google Calendars to plan my schedule, and always factor in my workouts a week ahead, so that I know when I will have time to exercise. I do this because it makes me feel physically better to exercise regularly, but I also notice a difference in how I feel mentally if I don't work out. From a financial perspective, I also want to make sure that I am getting the most out of my gym membership!

I schedule my food shopping trips in advance, too! This means that I am certain to have enough time to do a proper shop, rather than having to rush and not get everything I need. As with my menu planning, food shopping has become a bit of a ritual. I know, that sounds a bit strange, but hear me out! I plan to do my shopping in the early evening when my son is at a club and most people are at home eating their dinner, so the shops are quiet. I go alone and use it as an opportunity to enjoy some quiet time to myself. It is one of the only times in my week where I am not either talking to other people or listening to podcasts through my headphones. I take my time and feel grateful for the opportunity to spend time preparing for a healthy week ahead. When I get home, I organise everything as I put it away, wiping out the fridge before I fill it with the new food I have bought, and recycling any excess packaging. I know that food shopping can be dull, monotonous and can seem like a chore you'd rather not do, but by altering your mindset you can learn to enjoy it and see it as an influential and integral part of your journey towards weight loss and better health.

It can take a while to find what really works for you. Remember that you want your actions, routines, and outcomes to feel good each day, but also to be sustainable for the long term. Whatever you do going forward needs to be sustainable and manageable for the foreseeable future. Small, consistent changes which prove easy for you to stick to are the best way to proceed. I mentioned earlier in the book about my new habit of drinking a glass of lemon water with Celtic salt every morning. I do this every day now, even when I am away from home, because it is quick, easy, manageable, and aligned. On the contrary,

I have previously tried to commit to doing yoga every morning but there were more days where I didn't practice than those when I did! This was because committing to do something every single day amidst a busy lifestyle and plenty of other scheduled workouts was unrealistic and unsustainable. A better idea for me would be to commit to practising yoga twice a week, as this is something I could sustain, and feel good about achieving rather than pressured.

Task:

Journal around the following:

1. **What does balance mean to you?**

2. **How are you consistent in your life currently?**

3. **How do you think you could be more consistent when it comes to your health and fitness?**

4. **How do you allow yourself to be flexible with your food and fitness?**

Strategy Summary:

- It is essential to think long term. You can make changes along the way, but weight maintenance and being healthy is a journey that will last for as long as you are alive.
- Flexibility is important, as things happen, and life can change.
- Consistency is a commitment to doing the things that make you feel good most of the time.
- Sustainability is essential to lasting success.
- Balance is different for everyone. It's not transactional, but instead involves finding a way of life that feels natural and aligned for you and your family.
- Meal planning, exercise scheduling, scheduling your food shopping trips, and making small consistent changes are all things that can help with your creation of a long-term healthy lifestyle.

STRATEGY 19: CHOOSE YOUR PAIN.

"Everyone must choose one of two pains: the pain of discipline or the pain of regret" (Jim Rohn).

Being overweight is a pain, being fit and healthy is a pain! In all honesty, *any* decision you make in life comes with an element of pain, discomfort, hard work, or time and effort. Choosing to be self-employed may afford you freedom in when you work, but can also involve a much higher level of responsibility when compared to working for someone else. Living in a rural village offers you a calmer pace of life, and a sense of community, but also requires extra financial and time commitment in terms of getting out and about. Holidaying abroad might cost more and involve going to more effort during the booking process, but as a result you will be immersed in different cultures and have the opportunity to enjoy some sunshine! Travelling in your home country is often cheaper, quicker, and easier, but may feel limited in terms of the experience you have from your holiday. Life is a series of choices, and you must make the decisions that feel best and most aligned with your own situation and preferences. When it comes to health and fitness, I personally choose to exercise, eat a balanced diet, and live a healthy lifestyle. Even though those choices involve additional effort, time, money and sometimes doing things that it would be easy not to do, that is preferable to me in comparison to the feeling of being heavier and suffering with potential health problems. Decide to upgrade your problems. Recognise how much of a pain it is to weigh more than you would like to, and choose to swap that pain for the alternative 'pain', which may involve investing in a gym membership, taking the time to exercise, spending more time cooking, and choosing balanced meals over quick and tempting fast food. Reframing your health and weight situation in this way illustrates how a simple mindset change can help you to take ownership of your journey going forward. In this moment, you are asking yourself to make a decision about which reality feels worse to you – the one in which you remain overweight and feeling unhealthy, or the one where you swap that uncomfortable place for a place which will initially feel equally as uncomfortable, but will help you to lose weight and feel better eventually.

I really like the 'choose your pain' method, and I use it in day to day life to give me a push when I feel unmotivated. Picture this...I'm home late, rushing to cook dinner and I'm desperate to sit down and relax after I've eaten. But there are dishes by the sink and the kitchen is a bit of a mess. I have to choose my pain in that moment – postpone my relaxation time, do the dishes, and give the kitchen a quick clean there and then, even though I'm tired and don't really want to do it, or leave it until the morning, when I will wake up and wish I had done it the previous evening. Not only will this start my day off negatively, but the dishes are likely to be harder to wash if food has dried on to them, and the kitchen would have been easier to clean the night before. I'll almost *always* choose to do the dishes there and then, that same night. This is a trait I have had to develop over time – I haven't always been this way! I'm pleased that I approach choices in this way, but ultimately by inviting yourself to 'choose your pain', you are in complete control of how you live and how you react in times where there is a decision to be made. Knowing how the obesity rates in the UK have increased over recent years, I can only assume that for many people the prospect of doing what it takes to lose weight and be healthier is a version of 'hard' that they don't want to choose. I feel it is necessary to caveat that there are many other reasons why a person may struggle to lose weight or maintain a weight loss, including illness or disability, confusion over what to do for the best, and limited financial budget. Not everyone *easily* has the option to choose the healthy version, but it can be achieved with desire and determination.

Task:

Get out your diary and journal on the questions below.

What feels hard to you about weighing more than you would like to? Write down as many things as you can think of.

What feels hard to you about the process of losing weight?

In the short term, which feels harder – being overweight or doing what it takes to lose weight?

In the long term, over the next 20-30 years, which feels harder, being overweight or maintaining the weight you have lost?

Which version of 'hard' do you feel called to commit to right now?

Strategy Summary:

- Life brings a continuous stream of decisions – you must make your choices based on what feels best for you and your circumstances.
- The reality is that the outcomes of most decisions come with an element of difficulty or pain. You just have to decide which pain you prefer. Which is the lesser of two evils for you?
- It can be helpful to think about the short-term and long-term effects of choosing to work at being healthy and lose weight or choosing to remain as you are.
- You can use the 'choose your pain' strategy in many areas of life where more than one option is available to you. The concept can help motivate you to make choices which may be harder right now but make life easier in the long run.

STRATEGY 20: START WHERE YOU ARE BUT TAKE ACTION NOW.

"The best time to plant a tree was 50 years ago. The next best time is now". (Chinese proverb).

"Prevention is better than cure" – a sentiment I truly believe in and can relate to many areas of life. Keeping your house clean, tidy, and well-maintained stops it from falling into a state of disrepair and is easier than having to remedy issues after they have occurred. Bringing in your garden furniture and keeping it stored in a dry garage prevents it from getting wet and eventually going rotten or fabric getting mildew. Working on your relationship with your significant other consistently from the beginning is preferable to allowing circumstances to deteriorate and then needing to have counselling to try to save the relationship. This also applies to health and weight loss. In fact, when it comes to the nationwide struggle with weight and health, I strongly believe that the only way to change the trajectory for the future is to utilise the idea of 'prevention is better than cure'. Avoiding weight gain in the first place is much easier than trying to lose weight that has been gained, and maintaining health is easier than attempting to rid yourself of a health condition once it has taken hold. Having spent many years helping women who are already struggling with their weight and health, it has become very apparent to me just how hard these ladies must work to be able to lose weight and become healthier. Often, it just doesn't happen for them, despite their best efforts. The best possible way to tackle to this nationwide struggle would be to break the cycle of obesity and poor health *before* it can take negative effect. To do this, I think it would be necessary to work with parents and parents-to-be to support them in raising their children with positive eating habits, good relationships with food, and overall healthy, balanced lifestyles, thus preventing as many problems as possible from happening. This is the ideal scenario, but of course, this would only help very young children, and those who have not yet been born. It would take decades of working in this way to make a difference to the health of our society in general. I have worked with clients who are in their 50s, 60s and 70s, and have spent much of their adult life trying to lose weight, struggling, suffering, and in some cases, committing the best part of their lives to weight loss. I'll be honest - this makes me feel so sad! Now, of course, if you are reading this book, the chances are that you are not looking to prevent weight gain and poor health, but are, in fact, needing to address the problems you are already experiencing. I want to meet you where you are and help you to realise that the best time to break the cycle and start improving your health is *right now*, whatever age you are. Prevention *is* better than cure, but 'cure' is better than doing nothing at all! Going back to those examples at the beginning of this paragraph, if you have left your garden furniture outside for too long, eventually cleaning it up is better than letting it stay outside, becoming completely unusable. The same goes for the relationship – you may not have put in the effort that was needed to prevent issues from arising, but realising this, going to counselling and working on improving things is better than allowing things to get worse and worse, and both partners becoming increasingly unhappy. The earlier you can intervene in any situation, the better. If you are older and have struggled with your weight and health throughout your adulthood, you may wonder if some of the information in this book has any relevance to you. You may feel that it is too late to make a change. However, I want you to approach your weight loss and health improvement journey with an attitude of 'starting right now is better than starting 5, 10, or 20 years down the line'. If you start to make changes to your lifestyle now, improve your health, alter your mindset, and lose some weight, you will benefit far more than if you wait for another decade or two. The earlier you can begin, the better.

Do you have children or grandchildren? Do you plan to start a family in the future? If so, the 'prevention is better than cure' attitude may well enable you to help younger generations to reduce the struggling and suffering they might experience when it comes to weight and health. By changing how you think, eat, and live now, you can positively influence the children and grandchildren you have now, and any you have in the future. I love the idea that in 20 years my grandchildren could be benefitting from the way I have raised my son.

We all eat the same. Ever since my son had his very first meal at the age of 7 months we have always all eaten the same. His first experience of solid food was salmon, potato, and broccoli. Of course, I would make adaptations according to his developmental stage and his flavour preferences, for example, mashing some foods with a fork, cutting foods up into smaller pieces, and adding less spice to a curry to make it more enjoyable for him. There are certain foods and meals that Cassius doesn't like, such as steak or cheese and biscuits, and on the occasions that we are planning to have those, we will happily offer an alternative – he usually asks for fish! Because of how Cassius has been raised, he has not been used to eating foods that are specifically designed for children – think baby rice, pureed baby food, lunchbox foods, squeezy tubes of sweetened yoghurt, bear shaped ham slices, turkey dinosaurs...the list goes on! He is used to eating whole foods and adult meals, so there will be no need for him to transition between a child's diet and an adult one. His favourite foods include seafood, olives, halloumi, and mango. People are often surprised when they realise what Cassius will eat, and they will ask how I have managed to get him to eat such a range of foods without fuss. This wasn't difficult, it just involved limiting ultra-processed foods from the very start and offering as much variety as possible – basically the same recommendations as I've made for you in this book!

We have a healthy culture in our house. We take pride in being healthy and we practice what we preach when it comes to food, exercise, and lifestyle. We model the behaviour we'd like to see. We discuss nutrition and health honestly and openly with Cassius, and as a result, he is interested in where his food comes from, and how food and lifestyle can affect health.

We enjoy and share food – one of our favourite ways to eat is to serve food as a sharing platter or buffet. If we eat out, we hardly ever order our own separate meals. In fact, Cassius has only ever had a children's meal once in the seven years he has been eating solid food, as we usually order food to share between us – from the 'adult menu'! As a family, we love cooking, sitting down at the table for mealtimes, and taking time to enjoy our food.

My suggestions for how to raise children with healthy attitudes towards food may be useful to your own situation, but even if this does not apply to your life right now, reading my recommendations can help you to understand potential reasons for your own weight gain, and how society has ended up with such a problem with obesity and poor health. The more deeply you can understand, the easier your journey will be.

Going back to you, and how you can use the 'prevention is better than cure' concept, let's put aside any struggles that you've had in the past for now and focus on the future. Whatever you currently weigh, it is possible for you to prevent any further weight gain. Whatever your health situation, it is possible for you to work at preventing any conditions from getting worse. For example, if you know that you eat a lot of sugary foods but have not been diagnosed with diabetes, this is something to be celebrated, and an area where you can use the 'prevention is better than cure' mentality. You can feel fortunate that you have not reached that place yet, and don't have to take medication or attend regular check-ups with health professionals. You are not *yet* suffering from any of the negative symptoms of having diabetes. You can work to try to prevent this from happening. Even if you are diabetic, you can take action now to prevent things from getting worse. Wherever you are right now with your weight and health, you can aim to prevent things from worsening with the help of this book. The best time for you to start is right now. Start right where you are.

"Slowly is the fastest way to get to where you want to be".

I encourage you to create your healthy balanced lifestyle at your own pace, making small changes rather than attempting to alter everything at once. The bigger the change, the less likely you are to stick with it. Consistency is key as you embark on this journey.

What is the smallest thing that you could do *right now* to get you started on your weight loss journey? If you know that you want to join a gym, you need to visit a few, find out about membership types and costs, choose the one you prefer, sign up and book an induction. But your *first* action could be to take some time to research gyms in your area. Search online for information, look at websites, check out social media reviews, and ask friends and family for their opinions. Once you have completed this, you can then move on to enquiring for more information or contacting to book a visit. Other examples could be ordering a book if you know that you want to improve your knowledge on a particular area of health and nutrition, downloading an informative podcast to listen to on the drive to work tomorrow, making a template of a menu plan which you can then print off every week, or deciding on a set bed time and wake up time in order to improve your sleep. Returning to Atomic Habits for back up on this, James Clear says that 'too often, we convince ourselves that massive success requires massive action. Whether it is losing weight, building a business, writing a book, winning a championship, or achieving any other goal, we put pressure on ourselves to make some earth-shattering improvement that everyone will talk about'. Starting small is the easiest way to start, and it is more likely that you will succeed in your small change, continue to improve, and ultimately experience the outcomes you wanted.

I could suggest many more ideas to help you to begin changing your eating habits, exercise regime, and health, but I truly believe that you need to start with actions that reflect your own current situation, knowledge, and mindset. Some of you may be ready to join a gym, others may need to pluck up the courage to put their trainers on and go for a walk, or may feel more comfortable exercising at home. Likewise, when it comes to nutrition, you may be interested in my recommendations for books and podcasts on subjects like hormonal health, the effects of lectins, and how certain gene mutations can affect your health. Or, you may be at the stage where you need to learn more about why you should be limiting ultra-processed foods and eating plenty of good fats.

Start right where you are.

Task:

Q: What is the smallest thing you can do right now to kickstart your weight loss or improve your health? Choose something which feels good to you and is manageable right now. Go and complete that task.

Q: How did it feel doing the thing that you had chosen?

Q: How do you feel about your journey ahead now that you have started where you are and completed that one thing?

Strategy Summary:

- Prevention is better than cure in many areas, including health and weight management. I also believe that where prevention is no longer possible, 'cure' is better than doing nothing at all!
- The best way to work on reducing the high obesity statistics in the UK would be to work with parents to intercept the cycle, meaning that their children were less likely to struggle with their weight.
- The next best thing is to start right where you are!
- Approaching healthy eating as a family and adopting a healthy culture in your household are great ways to encourage your children to have a positive relationship with food.
- Even if you feel it's too late for you to benefit from these ideas, you may be able to use them to help your children, future children, or grandchildren. At the very least this strategy may help you to understand more about the journey that got you to a place where you weigh more than you would like to.
- Start with the smallest change you can make and do it now.

ALIGNING, MAINTAINING, AND EVOLVING

It has taken me eighteen years to really discover that the health and wellbeing magic happens when nutrition, movement, lifestyle, and mindset come into alignment. When it does, it all starts to feel more natural and as though everything is becoming easier. This alignment *must* happen for this to work for you, otherwise you will just feel as though you are on another diet. To get the most out of this book, master the advice and recommendations I have given you, and take additional time to work on those which don't happen on your first attempt. The journey ahead of you has no timeframe. Because you are now living a healthy lifestyle rather than following a diet, there is no end point. There is no need for perfection. You will go through periods of realignment, maintenance, and evolution – altering your nutrition, exercise habits and daily routines to fit your changing lifestyle, maintaining the results and outcomes you have achieved, and evolving in your knowledge and beliefs.

As we come to the end of this book, I want to leave you with some final encouragement to help you to live the life The Honest Weigh...the way that will help you to lose weight, maintain your weight when you reach a place that feels great, and live your happiest, healthiest life. When you commit to ditching diets for good, and realise that a long-term healthy lifestyle is the only way to sustainably manage your weight and your health, you will arrive at a place which gives you more freedom and contentment than you ever could have imagined. I am here in that place right now and have been for several years, but I will continue to develop within the nutrition and health world, expanding my knowledge and passion, and implementing whatever feels best for me and my health as I move through the years ahead of me. I have the rest of my life to enjoy the wonderful journey of looking after my health and feeling as amazing as possible. How lucky am I to have this privilege?! I want *you* to perceive weight loss, health, fitness, and wellbeing in this way too. Put the effort in but allow it to come naturally. Adapt and evolve as you change and as life changes. Make little tweaks and changes when you feel they are needed and have fun along the way. Aim to feel good consistently. Look back in a few months or years and notice how much better life is without dieting. Make your health and happiness your biggest priority, and love living this life for the *rest* of your life.

ABOUT THE AUTHOR

Gemma Mullinger

Gemma has been a qualified health and fitness professional for over a decade, with qualifications in Personal Training, Fitness Instructing, Yoga and Life Coaching. She is currently studying for a Masters in Human Nutrition at The University of Plymouth. Gemma's mission is to help as many people as possible to ditch the diets, lose weight, love food, and live their healthiest, happiest lives. Gemma lives in Cornwall with her son Cassius and loves geeking out on anything health related, cooking, sharing food with loved ones, camping, paddleboarding, cold water swimming, adventuring, reading, writing and fitness.

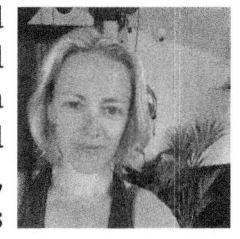

Instagram: @nutritiongems
LinkedIn: Gemma Mullinger

Printed in Dunstable, United Kingdom